Weight Watchers Freestyle Cookbook 2021

Affordable Tasty WW Freestyle Recipes to Lose Weight Fast and Never Let It Back, Be Healthy and Have a Happy Lifestyle

By Dr. Jenny Green

Introduction

I wish to personally congratulate you and thank you for purchasing this book: *"**Weight Watchers Freestyle Cookbook 2021- Affordable Tasty WW Freestyle Recipes to Lose Weight Fast and Never Let It Back, Be Healthy and Have a Happy Lifestyle**"*.

A large percentage of people around the world are overweight and they struggle to lose weight is real. You have probably heard tons of different advice on the Internet on how to lose weight. Thousands of books on dieting and exercising on the market. But did any of it work? Probably not. Some weight loss methods and diets require too much time or too much effort.

Then there are the diets and weight loss advice that just doesn't work. A lot of the crash diets and instant weight loss secrets can actually be damaging to your body and overall health. So, it's understandable why some people are unsuccessful at losing weight. Luckily for you, this book introduces the easy Weight Watchers diet which will work for anyone who is willing to give it a shot.

The diet includes pasta, steak, fried chicken, cheeseburger, ice cream, cookies, vegetables... yes, you can eat just about anything on Weight Watchers. Weight Watchers works by a point system which is geared to help you make healthier food decisions and encourage physical activity, so you can lose weight permanently. Weight Watchers technically isn't a diet, it's more of a lifestyle-change program.

This Weight Watchers Instant Pot Cookbook will allow you to learn to make some of the most delicious meals on the planet and more. It includes all sorts of recipes and the cooking instructions for preparing those amazing dishes. The Smart Points value and recipe nutrition are also given for every recipe as well. We have done our very best to include a diverse set of recipes to please everyone. Here you will find meals ready to be served for **breakfast, lunches, dinner, and for beans and grains, beef and pork, lamb, chicken, duck, fish and seafood, vegetables, and side dishes, soups and stews, poultry, and desserts**. Just about everything you can think of.

This book will open a new world of incredibly delicious and healthy foods to you. Use this book daily as it contains tons of healthy and incredibly tasty recipes that will satisfy your stomach and help you lose weight.

Thanks again for reading the book, I hope that you will enjoy it!

Table of Contents

Chapter 1: Essentials About the Weight Watchers Freestyle Program

Want to lose weight and still enjoy all your favorite foods? Then attempt on the Weight Watchers Freestyle Program. In this chapter, you will learn everything about Weight Watchers and how you can get started.

Brief History of the Weight Watchers Program

The history of the Weight Watchers program is easy to follow.

In early 1961, American business entrepreneur and co-founder of the Weight Watchers organization, Jean Nidetch had struggled with weight for most of her life and gone through every crazy diet out there where the weight was always coming back.

She gathered friends and members to her apartment every week to discuss their tips, achievements, and journey on losing weight. She later established a point system for foods to keep track of. This way dieters can focus eating more lean protein, fruits and vegetables and less sugar and saturated fat to lose weight.

By the end of 1962, Jean had lost more than 32 kilograms and many other participants shared similar results undergoing this program.

In 1962, the company Weight Watchers was founded and has grown immensely. The Weight Watchers program has attracted many celebrities such as Oprah Winfrey, Jessica, Simpson and Mariah Carey.

To this day, the Weight Watchers program has helped millions of people around the globe achieve their weight loss goals.

Advantages and Disadvantages of the Weight Watchers Diet

Weight Watchers is a widely popular and successful weight-loss program that has helped millions of people around the globe. But that doesn't necessarily mean it's right for everyone. It's essential you take a look at all the advantages and disadvantages of the Weight Watchers program before you commit.

Advantages of Weight Watchers

Here are some reasons why the diet plan may be the best route to help you lose weight.

- **No restrictions on food:** There is no official list of foods to avoid on Weight Watchers like you'll see on other diets. Instead, you track SmartPoints and garner FitPoints. The point system encourages you to eat more healthy foods such as fruits and vegetables while also enjoying your favorite sweets occasionally.
- **Nutritional value tips, cooking advice, recipes, and lifestyle changes are offered:** When you attend Weight Watchers meetings, meeting leaders is inclined to share effective nutritional advice with participants, for example, discussing the importance of adding more vegetables, healthy fats, low-fat dairy, reduced sugar, and drinking plenty of water to your diet.
- **The program is eligible for kids:** Some Weight Watchers locations hold meetings open for children. Teens as young as 13-years-old can participate in the Weight Watchers program if they have physician approval.
- **Slow and steady weight loss:** If you choose to commit to this program, you can expect to lose 1 to 2 pounds per week. You might lose even more when you first begin. Losing weight at a slow and steady rate makes weight loss more stable.
- **The program encourages portion control:** In order to keep track and record your SmartPoints you will need to measure your portions and serving sizes. Being able to control your portions will benefit you beyond Weight Watchers.
- **The program encourages exercise:** The Weight Watchers program encourages daily exercise which earns you FitPoints. Earning FitPoints will balance out your food intake.
- **You will cook at home:** You are more likely to eat healthy foods if you prepare them yourself at home. Weight Watchers offers recipes using your Instant Pot to help you learn how to prepare healthy meals.

Disadvantages of Weight Watchers

While Weight Watchers is a perfect solution for many to lose weight, it may not be appropriate for you. Take a look at the disadvantages of the Weight Watchers program.

- **Weight Watchers can be pricey:** The monthly cost for joining the Weight Watchers program will vary based on the level you choose, but if you have a substantial amount of weight to lose, the investment may be costly.
- **Group meetings aren't for everyone:** Some people prefer to keep their personal health and weight loss information private. You are not required to talk at Weight Watchers meetings. But Weight Watchers meetings are what makes the program special. However, if you prefer to avoid meetings, there are other options.
- **Weekly weigh-ins are a must:** Weighing yourself once a week to track your progress on the Weight Watchers program is a requirement. For some participants, this can be uncomfortable. For others, it keeps them motivated.
- **Weekly progress may discourage you:** Weekly progress checks can vary. Some weeks you will lose little weight. Sometimes you may even gain weight, even if you're doing everything right. This can discourage you from remaining in the program.
- **Keeping track of SmartPoints:** Keeping track of all the SmartPoints can be tedious and time-consuming.
- **Freedom to eat:** The Weight Watchers diet don't have any restrictions and you can eat almost anything you want. This freedom to eat anything you want can be too tempting. For some participants, diets that offer strict eating guidelines prove more effective.

Key Principles of Successful Weight Watchers and How It Works

Weight Watchers is an effective program because it's not really a diet. There are no specific restrictions on food intake, you just pay careful attention to portion sizes and keep track of SmartPoints.

Weight Watchers is less strict than many other diets – but the results are still promising, with participants able to lose up to 2- 4 pounds per week. This program still follows the three key principles: **Keep track of what you eat using SmartPoints, make healthy habits, and join a support group.**

Joining Weight Watchers, you learn how to calculate the number of SmartPoints to achieve your health and weight loss goals. Your daily and weekly SmartPoints allowance will be different depending on each person's status. After you are given a personalized SmartPoint limit, you get to decide which foods to eat based on the SmartPoints value appointed to each meal. No foods are banned on the program, the only rule is not to go over your SmartPoints allowance. _Foods that are nutritious,_ *healthy, and filling tend to have fewer SmartPoints, while high-fat, and high-carb meals tend to have larger SmartPoints value.*

This plan gives you the opportunity to choose healthy foods over the unhealthy ones. Some dieters even combine Weight Watchers with other diets such as the low-carb diet. It also means dieters won't have a hard time adopting this diet. You can follow the plan right this very second and it pretty much won't affect your day to day living.

The objective is to make better health decisions and lose weight in an unintimidating manner. It also heavily encourages including exercise and joining a support group. You are welcome to track your physical activity and exercise through activity trackers such as Fitbit. Here you will look at what exercise you are doing and how it will fit alongside your diet.

The third principle is joining a support group where you can meet like-minded people who share similar goals. You will also have a success coach watching over you who have been on the same journey as you. This is essential for the Weight Watchers program, and statistically, the more you attend the meetings, the higher your chance of weight loss success.

Weight Watchers: Foods You Can Eat

One reason why Weight Watchers Program is so popular is that there is no official restriction on what you can eat. The main objective of Weight Watchers is to keep track of your SmartPoints which helps control what you eat to lose weight.

Zero-point foods are foods that are low in saturated fat, sugar, carb, and calorie content. You should eat zero points foods as much as you can to help you lose weight, control your hunger, and stick with the Weight Watchers program. Here is the complete list of zero points foods which can help you make healthier food choices.

- Apples
- Unsweetened applesauce
- Apricots
- Arrowroots
- Artichoke hearts
- Artichokes
- Arugula
- Asparagus
- Bamboo shoots
- Banana
- Adzuki beans
- Black beans
- Green beans
- Chickpeas
- Great Northern beans
- Kidney beans
- Lima beans
- White beans
- Soybeans

- Navy beans
- Beets
- Berries
- Blackberries
- Blueberries
- Broccoli
- Brussel sprouts
- Green cabbage
- Red cabbage
- Bok choy
- Calamari
- Cantaloupe
- Carrots
- Cauliflower
- Caviar
- Celery
- Swiss chard
- Cherries
- Ground chicken breast
- Chicken breast or tenderloin
- Coleslaw mix
- Collards
- Corn
- White corn
- Cranberries
- Cucumber
- Daikon
- Dates
- Dragon fruit
- Egg substitutes
- Egg whites
- Eggplant
- Whole eggs
- Endive
- Fennel
- Figs
- Anchovies
- Sea Bass
- Carp
- Catfish

- Butterfish
- Cod
- Eel
- Haddock
- Halibut
- Herring
- Mackerel
- Monkfish
- Rainbow trout
- Rockfish
- Roe
- Salmon
- Sardines
- Seabass
- Striped mullet
- Swordfish
- Tuna
- Whitefish
- Tilapia
- Fruit cocktail
- Unsweetened fruit cup
- Fruit salad
- Unsweetened fruit
- Garlic
- Ginger root
- Grapefruit
- Grapes
- Honeydew melon
- Jackfruit
- Jerk chicken breast
- Kiwifruit
- Leeks
- Lemon
- Lemon zest
- Lentils
- Lettuce
- Lime
- Lime zest
- Mangoes
- Melon
- Brown mushrooms

- Button mushrooms
- Cremini mushrooms
- Italian mushrooms
- Portabella mushrooms
- Shiitake mushrooms
- Okra
- Onions
- Oranges
- Blood oranges
- Papayas
- Parsley
- Passionfruit
- Pears
- Peaches
- Peas
- Black-eyed peas
- Split peas
- Cayenne peppers
- Jalapeno peppers
- Poblano peppers
- Sweet bell peppers
- Pepperoncini
- Unsweetened pickles
- Pineapple
- Plumcots
- Plums
- Pomegranate seeds
- Pomegranate
- Pumpkin
- Pumpkin puree
- Radishes
- Radishes
- Raspberries
- Salsa verde
- Fat-free salsa

- Sauerkraut
- Scallions
- Seaweed
- Scallions
- Shallots
- Clams
- Crabs
- Crabmeat
- Crayfish
- Lobster
- Mussels
- Octopus
- Oysters
- Scallops
- Shrimp
- Squid
- Spinach
- Sprouts
- Summer squash
- Winter squash
- Zucchini
- Strawberries
- Tofu
- Tomatoes
- Tomato puree
- Tomato sauce
- Turkey
- Turnips
- Vegetable stick
- Mixed vegetables
- Water chestnuts
- Watermelon
- Greek yogurt
- Plain yogurt
- Soy yogurt

A Word of Caution on Zero Point Foods

Zero-point foods are the best thing about the Weight Watchers program but this may lead to slower weight loss. You should try to eat zero-point foods in moderation and only when you're hungry.

Do your best not to overeat and control your portion sizes even if it is zero-point foods. For example, while eggs are zero points, it isn't recommended to have an 8-egg omelet for breakfast.

Weight Watchers: Foods to Avoid

In the Weight Watchers, you should avoid foods with high SmartPoints value. *Food that are high in refined carbs and fats and low protein tend to have a higher point value in the Weight Watchers program.*

Such food items include cupcakes, cookies, ice cream, cheeseburgers, pasta, chili cheese fries, deep fried chicken, and cherry pies. Most foods served at fast food restaurants tend to have over 20 points! A triple whopper with cheese is 31 points!

So, what foods should you think twice on? Fast foods, junk foods, and sugary drinks are the absolute worst to eat if you want to feel satiated while cutting your caloric intake. This also includes many foods made with flour, gluten, or added sugar and most high-fat foods. These foods taste luxuriant but are loaded with fat and calories. Because of this, we eat them so fast that we eat too much before we feel satiated.

This doesn't mean you must cut all your favorite treats out of your diet entirely. Remember, you can eat anything on the Weight Watchers program, but only in moderation. Don't think you can eat a Bacon Cheeseburger Deluxe for lunch every day and expect to lose 2 pounds a week.

Chapter 2: Top Tips on Sticking with the Weight Watchers Freestyle Program

There are several useful strategies and advice that will help you get started on the Weight Watchers program. Below are top tips that will help you succeed in Weight Watchers:

Drink lots of water: Drinking water is essential for health, and it's going to help immeasurably in the Weight Watchers program. Drinking water also has many benefits including easier weight loss, clear skin, improved digestion, more energy, and increased mental clarity.

Learn portion control: Learning portion control is extremely important in Weight Watchers. You must be able to recognize ounces and cups when dining out or even cooking at home. If you can control portion and serving sizes, this can help ease the path to successful weight loss.

Don't overeat fruit: Fruits are zero SmartPoints food value because it is encouraged for dieters to eat them. They make good snacks and highly nutritious. So, don't be afraid to eat them. However, only eat fruit until you're satisfied, not full. It is recommended to eat only five servings of fruit per day.

Figure out your why: Motivation is crucial for weight loss. You will be more motivated to lose weight after you know why you want to lose weight in the first place. Some reasons include: having more energy, lowering your cholesterol, live longer, or look better. Find out why you committed to Weight Watchers program and remind yourself of it every day.

Don't guess SmartPoints: The most important thing to understand about SmartPoints is that you cannot guess SmartPoint values. The calculation of SmartPoints goes beyond calories. The calorie count you find on nutrition labels is based on the amount of energy in a food before it enters your body. After you consume it, your body processes it. As it processes the food, a portion of the food's calories is burned for body energy. SmartPoints are calculated based on the energy that is available after your body processed a food. This means you cannot just look at a food label and guess how much SmartPoints there is. You will over guess and throw the entire point system off balance.

Eat as many zero Points foods as you can: Take a look at the zero Points food list by Weight Watchers. There is plenty of tasty foods you can eat from and it's highly recommended to choose foods with zero points value whenever you can.

Don't cheat: If you want to eat something that is 9 points, and you only have 8 points left for the day, don't eat it believing it won't hurt you. It will really affect your body, diet, and mentality by adding that extra point. To find success in this program, you must be honest with yourself.

Share your journey: When you tell someone about your journey and progress, you are more likely to stay on track. You can participate in Weight Watchers meetings where you share your experience with other participants and leaders. You can even talk with someone, not on the diet, just someone who is supportive and makes you the most comfortable.

Plan your meals: By planning your meals ahead of time, it will help keep track of your SmartPoints throughout the day. If you're planning on dining out, figure out what you're going to order before you leave. If you're not a fan of meal prep, maybe you should start getting into the habit of it.

Track everything: Track your SmartPoints as you go. It's recommended that you carry a small notebook or have a tracking app on your phone. If you wait till before you sleep, you will probably forget some meals and snacks you had earlier today.

Don't forget exercise: Find ways to become more active and to move more in your life. When people lose weight through dieting, they tend to think that exercise is no longer necessary. They're wrong. You can lose weight quicker and become more fit if you include regular aerobic and cardio exercise in your life.

Expect progress, not perfection: Don't set yourself up for failure by seeking perfection. Don't set impossible goals. As you start the Weight Watchers program, you will go through days where you feel unmotivated and see no progress and you will go through days where you feel like you're on top of the world.

Be patient with yourself: While other diets may be too strict or just not working, the Weight Watchers program does work but it takes time to notice significant results. Remember, the Weight Watchers program is more of a lifestyle change than a diet. You won't find overnight success joining this program. You must be patient with yourself and not fight the change.

Eat high water content fruits and vegetables: If you can't drink a big jug of water, try eating high water content fruits and vegetables instead. Below you will find a list of high water content fruit and veggies.

Fruit and water content:

- Watermelon, 92% water content
- Strawberry, 92% water content

- Grapefruit, 91% water content
- Cantaloupe, 90% water content
- Peach, 88% water content
- Pineapple, 87% water content
- Cranberry, 87% water content
- Orange, 87% water content
- Raspberry, 87% water content
- Apricot, 86% water content
- Blueberry, 85% water content
- Plum, 85% water content
- Apple, 84% water content
- Pear, 84% water content
- Cherry, 81% water content
- Grape, 81% water content
- Banana, 74% water content

Veggies and water content:

- Cucumber, 96% water content
- Lettuce, 96% water content
- Zucchini, 95% water content
- Radish, 95% water content
- Celery, 95% water content
- Tomato, 94% water content
- Green cabbage, 93% water content
- Cauliflower, 92% water content
- Eggplant, 92% water content
- Red cabbage, 92% water content
- Pepper, 92% water content
- Spinach, 92% water content
- Broccoli, 91% water content
- Carrots, 87% water content
- Green pea, 79% water content
- Potato, 79% water content

Keep a Weight Watchers diary: Studies show that Weight Watchers participants who don't keep a food diary have a tougher time losing weight. It is recommended that you keep daily food records to successfully follow the Weight Watchers program and maintain steady weight loss.

I want you to find success with your health and your weight loss journey. In order to achieve this, you must follow the Weight Watchers program, but learn how to modify your entire way of thinking. The tips above will help you find ultimate success in your physical, mental, and financial health journey.

If you want to learn more dieting tips, look at WeightWatchers.com community message boards.

Chapter 3: Everything About Weight Watchers Free Style SmartPoints

The Weight Watchers program is based on a SmartPoint system which tracks the food you eat. This system encourages dieters to choose highly nutritious and healthy foods rather than junk food. In this chapter, you will learn everything you need to know about Weight Watchers Freestyle SmartPoints.

What are SmartPoints and How Does It Work?

SmartPoints is a revitalization of the counting ProPoint system that is quite easy to understand.

SmartPoints encourages you to make nutritious, healthier informed food decisions so that you choose food that make you feel better, have more energy and lose weight as opposed to unhealthy food. Hence, the reason why they are called SmartPoints.

With SmartPoints, foods that are greater in sugar and saturated fat have higher SmartPoints values. Foods with more lean protein lower the SmartPoints value. This directs you towards healthier food decisions.

Every food, every meal, every recipe has their own SmartPoints value that is based on calories, sugar, protein, and saturated fat. The more protein decreases the SmartPoints value while saturated fat and sugar increase the SmartPoints value.

How does it work?

When you join the Weight Watchers program, you will be given a customized SmartPoints budget which is influenced by your current weight, height, gender, and age.

SmartPoints also have a daily allowance, in addition to a weekly allowance to use on splurges, cravings, or larger portions. It's also easy to keep track of your SmartPoints value which in return allow you to make healthier and more gratifying food decisions.

Healthy eating habits that work best for you.

Counting SmartPoints you can eat anything you like – nothing is off limits. You will be losing weight by eating tasty foods that fill you up. Using this system gives you the freedom and flexibility to enjoy your food preferences and lose weight.

Example Calculation of SmartPoints

We want to help you calculate Weight Watchers SmartPoints so you can enjoy all sorts of food. In this section, you will learn how to calculate SmartPoints for your favorite dishes.

Before you begin the program, you will need to be aware of one small adjustment to the SmartPoints system. Weight Watchers is now focusing on other contents such as saturated fats and sugars. So, while a honeybun used to be 2 points, it will now be 6 points. This promotes more awareness of your food choices.

The new Weight Watchers program has a daily limit of 30 points rather than 26. So, this change makes you rethink reaching for a bowl of ice cream instead of fresh fruit.

How to Calculate Weight Watchers SmartPoints

The math behind Weight Watchers points is complicated to calculate unless you are a licensed nutritionist. I recommend you use an online Weight Watchers SmartPoints calculator.

Using an online calculator, you will need to provide the calories, saturated fats, sugar, and protein content that is found on the recipe nutrition label.

Site: http://www.calculatorcat.com/health/weight-watchers-calculator.html

How to Calculate Recipe Calories and Nutrition

Some nutrition analyzers you find online don't provide the proper information you in. The best in-depth calorie and nutrition calculator is VeryWellFit.com recipe analyzer.

You can enter practically any ingredient into the recipe analyzer and it gives you the full nutrition information for the whole recipe. Take note of calories, fats, sugar, and protein content

Take note of calories, fats, sugar, and protein per recipe and enter those numbers into the Calculator Cat tool above to figure out the total SmartPoints per recipe.

Divide that number by servings and you will have the SmartPoints value for literally any recipe you have.

Site: https://www.verywellfit.com/recipe-nutrition-analyzer-4157076

The two tools mentioned above will be a useful and effective tool to have in order to calculate recipes and nutrition information for your favorite foods and meals.

Remember to choose healthy foods with low Weight Watchers SmartPoints to find any success in this program.

Your Weight Loss Expectations

Healthy and permanent weight loss is achieved gradually, at a rate of no quicker than 2 pounds per week. The program follows this rule, where dieters can expect to lose 1 to 2 pounds per week on average. But, several factors can change this number. It is advisable to consult your physician or doctor before starting Weight Watchers.

Measuring weight loss

Fat loss main principle is to burn more calories than you consume to achieve weight loss. However, weight loss is much more complicated.

Weight is the force of gravity measured on a weighing scale. For example, weight yourself before and after a large meal and a few cups of water. You'll notice significant differences. For the most precise weight loss log, the Handbook of Obesity Treatment suggests it's best to weigh yourself at the same time of the day once per week without any clothes.

Factors in first-week weight loss

Many people lose more weight their first week on the Weight Watchers program than the weeks after.

This is primarily because of weight loss, caused by decreasing sodium intake and increasing your water intake.

Weight Watchers

Weight watchers cause weight loss by helping you reduce your calorie intake.

There are no restrictions on the Weight Watchers program. Instead, all foods are allowed but only in moderation.

The plan is designed to give an incentive to opt for low-fat, high fiber foods rather than high-fat, low-fiber foods. These foods are unprocessed and low in sodium. With this said, Weight Watchers dieters can expect to lose up to 2 pounds to 4 pounds during their first week following the program.

The Weight Watchers program was created to educate you on portion control to gradually lose weight and maintain a healthy body weight.

Don't freak out about how much weight you lost during any week, including your first week on the program. It can be tempting to give up if your first week didn't meet your expectations. Focus on making healthy food decisions and remember that permanent weight loss is a lifestyle change.

Chapter 4: Easy and Delicious Recipes with SmartPoints

Cooking and Culinary Units Conversion Chart

If you can quickly convert measurements of recipes, it will save you a ton of time.

The cooking conversion chart below can act as a quick reference list when you follow any of the cookbook's recipes.

Unit:	Equals:	Ounces:	Volume:	Weight:
Pinch	1/16 teaspoon	N/A	N/A	N/A
Dash	1/8 teaspoon	N/A	N/A	N/A
1 teaspoon	N/A	N/A	5 milliliters	N/A
1 tablespoon	3 teaspoons	1/3 ounce	15 milliliters	14.3 grams
1/8 cup	2 tablespoons	1 ounce	30 milliliters	28.3 grams
¼ cup	4 tablespoons	2 ounces	60 milliliters	56.7 grams
½ cup	8 tablespoons	4 ounces	120 milliliters	113.4 grams or ¼ pound
¾ cup	12 tablespoons	6 ounces	180 milliliters	
1 cup	16 tablespoons	8 ounces	240 milliliters	225 grams or ½ pound
1 pint	32 tablespoons or 2 cups	16 ounces	500 milliliters	450 grams or 1 pound
1 quart	4 cups or 2 pints	32 ounces	95 liter	N/A
1 gallon	16 cups or 4 quarts	128 ounces	3.79 liters	N/A

Pork, Beef and Lamb Recipes

1. <u>Full-Flavored Lamb and Winter Squash Tagine with Apricots</u>

Time: 50 minutes

Servings: 6

Freestyle SmartPoints: 6

Ingredients:

- 1 pound of lamb shoulders, cubed
- 1 tablespoon of coconut oil
- 1 onion, chopped
- 3 garlic cloves, minced
- 1-inch fresh ginger, grated
- ½ pound of medium-sized winter squash, seeded and cubed
- 2 to 3 cups of beef stock
- ¾ cup of dried apricots
- 1 (14-ounce) can of diced tomatoes
- 1 (14-ounce) can of chickpeas
- 1 teaspoon of salt
- 1 teaspoon of black pepper

Instructions:

- Press "Saute" function on your Instant Pot and add the coconut oil.
- Once the oil is hot, add the onions and cook until brown, stirring occasionally.
- Add the cubed lamb to the Instant Pot and cook until brown on all sides.
- Add the garlic and ginger. Give a good stir.
- Add the cubed squash, beef stock, dried apricots, diced tomatoes, chickpeas, salt, and pepper to the pot.
- Lock the lid and cook at high pressure for 20 minutes.
- When the cooking is done, quick release the pressure and remove the lid.
- Serve and enjoy!

Nutrition information per serving:

- Calories: 446
- Fat: 12.4g
- Carbohydrates: 48.4g
- Dietary Fiber: 13.5g
- Protein: 36g

2. <u>Good Tasting Pork Carnitas (Mexican Pulled Pork)</u>

Time: 1 hour and 20 minutes

Servings: 11

Freestyle SmartPoints: 3

Ingredients:

- 2 ½ pounds of trimmed, boneless pork shoulder, cut into 4 pieces
- 2 tablespoons of olive oil
- 1 cup of chicken broth
- 3 chipotle peppers in adobo sauce
- 2 bay leaves
- 2 tablespoons of garlic powder
- ¼ teaspoon of dry adobo seasoning
- ½ teaspoon of onion powder
- 1 ½ teaspoon of cumin
- ¼ teaspoon of dry oregano
- 2 teaspoons of salt
- 1 teaspoon of black pepper

Instructions:

- Season the pork shoulder with salt and pepper.
- Press "Saute" function and add the olive to the Instant Pot.
- Once the oil is hot, add the pork pieces and cook until brown on all sides, about 5 minutes. Remove and set aside.
- Season the pork with garlic powder, cumin, oregano, and dry adobo seasoning.
- Add the chicken broth, chipotle peppers, bay leaves, and pork to the Instant Pot.
- Lock the lid and cook at high pressure for 80 minutes.
- When the cooking is done, naturally release the pressure and remove the lid.
- Transfer the pork to a cutting board and shred using two forks. Return the shredded pork to the pot and stir into the liquid.
- Remove the bay leaves and adjust the seasoning as needed.
- Serve and enjoy!

Nutrition information per serving:

- Calories: 160
- Fat: 7g
- Carbohydrates: 1g
- Dietary Fiber: 1g
- Protein: 20g

3. <u>Magnificent Beef and Broccoli</u>

Time: 20 minutes   Servings: 6   Freestyle SmartPoints: 3

Beef Ingredients:

- 1 ½ pound of boneless beef chuck roast, thinly sliced
- 4 cups of broccoli florets
- 2 garlic cloves, minced
- ½ teaspoon of fresh ginger, grated
- 1 teaspoon of sesame oil
- 1 teaspoon of salt
- 1 teaspoon of black pepper

Sauce Ingredients:

- 1/3 cup of low-sodium soy sauce
- 2/3 cup of beef broth
- 2 tablespoons of oyster sauce
- 3 tablespoons of brown sugar
- 1 ½ teaspoon of sesame oil
- ¼ teaspoon of red pepper chili flake

Cornstarch Ingredients:

- 2 ½ tablespoons of cornstarch plus 3 tablespoons of water

Instructions:

- Season the beef chuck roast with salt, pepper, and sesame oil.
- Press "Saute" function on your Instant Pot and add the olive to the Instant Pot.
- Once the oil is hot, add the beef and cook for 2 minutes or until brown.
- Add the garlic and ginger and cook for 1 minute or until fragrant, stirring occasionally.
- In a medium bowl, add all the sauce ingredients until well combined. Pour the sauce over the beef.
- Lock the lid and cook at high pressure for 6 minutes.
- Meanwhile, in a bowl, add the broccoli and ¼ cup of water. Microwave for 2 to 3 minutes or until the broccoli is tender.
- When the timer beeps, quick release the pressure and remove the lid.
- Press "Saute" function on your Instant Pot and stir in the cornstarch mixture.
- Add the broccoli florets and cook until the sauce has thickened, stirring occasionally. Adjust the seasoning as needed. Serve and enjoy!

Nutrition information per serving:

- Calories: 475
- Fat: 31.9g
- Carbohydrates: 12.8g
- Protein: 32.8g

4. <u>Remarkable Cajun Chili</u>

Time: 30 minutes   Servings: 8   Freestyle SmartPoints: 4

Ingredients:

- 2 tablespoons of olive oil
- 1 green pepper, chopped
- 1 onion, chopped
- 2 celery ribs, chopped
- 2 garlic cloves, minced
- 1 pound of ground beef
- 2 links Andouille Sausage, sliced
- 7-ounces of raw shrimp, peeled and deveined
- 1 tablespoon of parsley, freshly chopped
- 2 ½ tablespoons of Cajun seasoning
- 1 (14-ounce) can of crushed tomatoes
- 1 (14.5-ounce) can of fire roasted tomatoes
- 1 (15-ounce) can of red kidney beans, drained and rinsed
- 2 tablespoons of tomato paste
- 1 teaspoon of salt
- 2 bay leaves

Instructions:

- Press "Saute" function and add 1 tablespoon of olive oil to your Instant Pot.
- Once the oil is hot, add the green pepper, onion, celery, and garlic. Cook for 4 minutes or until softened, stirring occasionally.
- Add the remaining 1 tablespoon of olive oil and ground beef. Cook until brown, stirring frequently.
- Add the sausage and cook for 5 minutes or until brown, stirring occasionally.
- Add the shrimp and remaining ingredients to your Instant Pot. Stir until well combined.
- Lock the lid and cook at high pressure for 10 minutes.
- When the cooking is done, naturally release the pressure and remove the lid.
- Press "Saute" function on your Instant Pot and cook for 5 to 7 minutes or until the chili has thickened, stirring occasionally. Serve and enjoy!

Nutrition information per serving:

- Calories: 344
- Fat: 16.4g
- Carbohydrates: 24g
- Dietary Fiber: 6.4g
- Protein: 27.6g

5. Phenomenal Chipotle Chili

Time: 40 minutes

Servings: 4

Freestyle SmartPoints: 5

Ingredients:

- 1 pound of ground beef
- 1 tablespoon of coconut oil
- 1 large onion, finely chopped
- 6 garlic cloves, minced
- 1 teaspoon of chipotle chili powder
- 1 tablespoon of red chili powder
- 1 teaspoon of oregano
- 1 teaspoon of cumin powder
- 2 chipotle chilies in adobo sauce, roughly chopped
- 2 cups of fresh tomatoes, chopped
- 1 cup of dried kidney beans, soaked overnight
- 1 cup of water or beef broth
- 1 teaspoon of salt
- 1 teaspoon of black pepper

Topping ingredients:

- Sliced avocados
- Crushed nachos
- Lime wedges
- Sour cream
- Cilantro
- Shredded cheddar cheese

Instructions:

- Press "Saute" function on your Instant Pot and add the coconut oil.
- Once the oil is hot and ready, add the ground beef and cook until brown, stirring occasionally.
- Add the onions and garlic. Cook until softened, stirring occasionally.
- Add the remaining ingredients to your Instant Pot and stir until well combined.
- Lock the lid and cook at high pressure for 30 minutes.
- When the cooking is done, naturally release the pressure and remove the lid.
- Stir in the chili and adjust the seasoning as needed.
- Spoon the chili into serving bowls and add desired toppings. Serve and enjoy!

Nutrition information per serving:

- Calories: 459
- Fat: 26g
- Carbohydrates: 25.4g
- Protein: 28g

6. <u>Homemade Hamburger Helper</u>

Time: 10 minutes

S rvings: 6

Freestyle SmartPoints: 7

Ingredients:

- 1 pound of ground beef
- 2 cups of beef broth
- 2 cups of elbow macaroni
- 1 cup of heavy cream
- 2 cups of shredded cheddar cheese
- ½ cup of shredded American cheese
- 1 tablespoon of onion powder
- 1 tablespoon of garlic powder

Instructions:

- Press "Saute' function on your Instant Pot and add the ground beef and seasonings. Cook until the meat is brown, stirring occasionally.
- Add the beef broth, elbow macaroni, and heavy cream to your Instant Pot.
- Lock the lid and cook at high pressure for 4 minutes.
- When the cooking is done, quick release the pressure and remove the lid.
- Stir in the cheddar cheese and American cheese. Continue to cook and stir until all the cheese has melted.
- Serve and enjoy!

Nutrition information per serving:

- Calories: 992
- Fat: 61g
- Carbohydrates: 61g
- Dietary Fiber: 2g
- Protein: 47g

7. Famous Spaghetti

Time: 15 minutes

Servings: 6

Freestyle SmartPoints: 5

Ingredients:

- 1 pound of lean ground beef
- ½ teaspoon of salt
- ½ teaspoon of garlic powder
- ½ teaspoon of onion powder
- ½ teaspoon of Italian seasoning
- 1 pound of spaghetti noodles, break in half
- 1 (24-ounce) jar of spaghetti sauce
- 4 ½ cup of water
- 1 (14.5-ounce) can of diced tomatoes

Instructions:

- Press "Saute" function on your Instant Pot and add the ground beef.
- Add the salt, garlic powder, onion powder, and Italian seasoning. Cook until the ground beef is completely brown, stirring occasionally.
- Turn off "Saute' function on your Instant Pot and discard any excess grease from the beef if necessary.
- Add the spaghetti noodles, spaghetti sauce, water, and diced tomatoes to your Instant Pot.
- Lock the lid and cook at high pressure for 8 minutes.
- When the cooking is done, quick release the pressure and remove the lid
- Stir the spaghetti and adjust the seasoning as needed. Serve and enjoy!

Nutrition information per serving:

- Calories: 689
- Fat: 7.7g
- Carbohydrates: 116.9g
- Dietary Fiber: 4.2g
- Protein: 38.9g

8. Tempting Beef Short Ribs

Time: 1 hour and 20 minutes

Servings: 10

Freestyle SmartPoints: 9

Ingredients:

- 4 pounds of boneless beef short ribs
- 2 tablespoons of olive oil
- 1 large onion, chopped
- 2 shallots, finely chopped
- 3 garlic cloves, minced
- 3 large carrots, chopped
- 1 sprig of rosemary
- 2 sprigs of thyme, leaves removed
- 1 cup of red wine
- 1 cup of chicken broth
- 3 tablespoons of balsamic vinegar
- 2 teaspoons of salt
- 1 teaspoon of black pepper

Instructions:

- Season the ribs with salt and pepper.
- Press "Saute" function on your Instant Pot and add 1 tablespoon of olive oil.
- Add the ribs to your Instant Pot and sear for 6 to 8 minutes.
- Flip the ribs and cook for 5 minutes or until brown.
- Once the meat is brown, transfer to a plate and add the remaining tablespoon of olive oil.
- Add the onions, shallots, garlic, and carrots to your Instant Pot and cook until soft.
- Add the red wine, chicken broth, and balsamic vinegar to your Instant Pot. Stir until well combined.
- Return the beef short ribs to your Instant Pot and top with rosemary.
- Lock the lid and cook at high pressure for 45 minutes.
- When the cooking is done, naturally release the pressure and remove the lid.
- Transfer the ribs to a serving platter.
- Press "Saute" function and bring the broth to a boil. Cook until half of the liquid has reduced and thickened, stirring occasionally. Sprinkle with thyme leaves
- Pour the sauce over the ribs. Serve and enjoy!

Nutrition information per serving:

- Calories: 407
- Fat: 14.3g
- Carbohydrates: 5.9g
- Dietary Fiber: 0.9g
- Protein: 56.2g

Chicken, Turkey and Duck Recipes

1. <u>Summer Italian Chicken</u>

Time: 30 minutes

Servings: 8

Freestyle SmartPoints: 3

Ingredients:

- 8 boneless, skinless chicken thighs
- 2 tablespoons of avocado oil
- 1 onion, chopped
- 2 medium carrots, chopped
- ½ pounds of cremini mushrooms stemmed and quartered
- 4 garlic cloves, minced
- 1 tablespoon of tomato paste
- 2 cups of cherry tomatoes
- ½ cup of green olives pitted
- ½ cup of fresh basil leaves, thinly sliced
- ¼ cup of Italian parsley, chopped
- 1 teaspoon of salt
- 1 teaspoon of black pepper

Instructions:

- Season the chicken thighs with salt and pepper.
- Press "Saute" function on your Instant Pot and add the avocado oil.
- Once the oil is hot, add the onions, carrots, and mushrooms. Cook for 3 to 5 minutes or until the vegetables have softened.
- Stir in the garlic and tomato paste. Cook for 30 seconds or until fragrant.
- Add the chicken, cherry tomatoes, green olives. Stir until well combined.
- Lock the lid and cook at high pressure for 8 minutes.
- When the cooking is done, quick release the pressure and remove the lid.
- Stir in the basil leaves and parsley. Adjust the seasoning as needed.
- Serve and enjoy!

Nutrition information per serving:

- Calories: 318
- Fat: 11.9g
- Carbohydrates: 7.1g
- Dietary Fiber: 2g
- Protein: 44.2g

2. Delectable Chicken Enchiladas

Time: 50 minutes   Servings: 4   Freestyle SmartPoints: 3

Ingredients:

- 1 pound of boneless, skinless chicken thighs
- 2 cups of ancho chili sauce
- ½ cup of onions, chopped
- 12 corn tortillas
- 3 tablespoons of olive oil
- ½ cup of crumbled queso fresco
- 2 cups of shredded Monterey Jack cheese
- 1 teaspoon of salt
- 1 teaspoon of black pepper

Instructions:

- Add the chicken thighs and ancho chili sauce to your Instant Pot.
- Lock the lid and cook at high pressure for 10 minutes.
- When the cooking is done, naturally release the pressure for 10 minutes and quick release any remaining pressure.
- Remove the lid and transfer the chicken to a large bowl. Shred the chicken using forks. Stir in 2/3 cup of the ancho chili sauce.
- Chop the onions and put into a small bowl.
- Preheat your oven to 350 degrees Fahrenheit.
- Place tortillas on a baking sheet and lightly brush with olive oil.
- Place inside your oven and bake for 3 minutes or until warm. Remove from the oven.
- Spoon ½ cup of the warm ancho chili sauce into a baking dish.
- Working one-by-one, lightly coat each tortilla with the sauce and generously add the shredded chicken and onions on the tortilla.
- Sprinkle shredded Monterey Jack cheese over the chicken and onion.
- Wrap the tortilla and repeat until all the tortillas are used up.
- Once all the tortillas are prepared, generously pour leftover ancho chili sauce over them and sprinkle remaining cheese over the enchiladas.
- Place inside your oven and bake for 8 to 10 minutes or until warmed through.
- Sprinkle crumbled queso fresco over the enchiladas. Serve and enjoy!

Nutrition information per serving:

- Calories: 695
- Fat: 38g
- Carbohydrates: 67g
- Protein: 51g

3. <u>Finger Licking Chicken Marsala</u>

Time: 40 minutes   Servings: 4   Freestyle SmartPoints: 4

Ingredients:

- 5 boneless, skinless chicken breasts, halved or thinly sliced
- ½ cup of all-purpose flour
- 3 tablespoons of butter
- 3 tablespoons of olive oil
- 1 cup of mushrooms, stemmed and halved
- 1 shallot, thinly sliced
- 3 garlic cloves, minced
- 2/3 cup of marsala wine
- 2/3 cup of chicken stock
- ½ cup of heavy cream
- 1 teaspoon of garlic powder
- 1 teaspoon of salt
- 1 teaspoon of black pepper

Instructions:

- Add the flour on a shallow plate and dredge the chicken breasts in the flour, shake off any excess flour.
- Press "Saute" function on your Instant Pot and add the 2 tablespoons of oil and 2 tablespoons of butter.
- Once the butter is melted, working in batches, add the chicken breasts and cook on both sides until golden. Set the cooked chicken aside.
- Add the remaining tablespoons of oil and butter to your Instant Pot.
- Add the mushrooms, shallots, and garlic. Cook for 5 minutes or until tender, stirring occasionally. Season with salt and pepper.
- Add the marsala wine and chicken stock to your Instant Pot. Stir until well combined. Lay the chicken on top of the mushrooms.
- Lock the lid and cook at high pressure for 10 minutes.
- When the cooking is done, naturally release the pressure for 5 minutes and quick release any remaining pressure. Remove the lid. Remove the chicken and set aside.
- Press "Saute" function and stir in the heavy cream. Stir until well combined. Cook for 5 minutes or until thickened, stirring occasionally.
- Return the chicken back to the pot and stir until well coated. Serve and enjoy!

Nutrition information per serving:

- Calories: 622
- Fat: 35g
- Carbohydrates: 23g
- Dietary Fiber: 1g
- Protein: 41g

4. <u>Award Winning Turkey Chili</u>

Time: 18 minutes   Servings: 8   Freestyle SmartPoints: 3

Ingredients:

- 1 ½ pound of ground turkey
- 8 bacon slices, chopped
- 1 (15-ounce) can of pinto beans, rinsed and drained
- 1 (15-ounce) can of black beans, rinsed and drained
- 1 (15-ounce) can of diced tomatoes, rinsed and drained
- 1 (6-ounce) can of tomato paste
- 1 small red onion, chopped
- 1 red bell pepper, chopped
- 1 orange bell pepper, chopped

- 1 jalapeno, minced
- 2 cups of chicken stock
- 1 tablespoon of dried oregano
- 1 teaspoon of ground cumin
- 2 teaspoons of salt
- 1 teaspoon of black pepper
- 1 teaspoon of smoked paprika
- 2 tablespoons of chili powder
- 1 tablespoon of Worcestershire sauce
- 1 tablespoon of garlic, minced

Topping Ingredients:

- Sour cream
- Cilantro

- Shredded cheese

Instructions:

- Press "Saute" function on your Instant Pot and add the bacon. Cook until brown and crispy, stirring occasionally. Remove the bacon and set on a paper towel-lined plate. Add the onions and peppers and cook until softened, stirring occasionally.
- Add the ground turkey and cook until browned, stirring occasionally.
- Add the remaining ingredients and cooked bacon. Stir until well combined.
- Lock the lid and cook at high pressure for 18 minutes.
- When the cooking is done, naturally release the pressure for 15 minutes and quick release any remaining pressure. Remove the lid.
- Ladle the chili into serving bowls and top with desired toppings. Serve and enjoy!

Nutrition information per serving:

- Calories: 286
- Fat: 11.7g
- Carbohydrates: 19.7g
- Dietary Fiber: 6.3g
- Protein: 26.3

5. **Tantalizing Beer-And-Mustard Pulled Turkey**

Time: 1 hour

Servings: 4

Freestyle SmartPoints: 6

Ingredients:

- 2 (1 ½ pound) bone-in, skinless turkey thighs
- 1 (12-ounce) bottle of dark beer
- ½ teaspoon of garlic powder
- 1 teaspoon of black pepper
- 1 teaspoon of salt
- 1 teaspoon of dry mustard
- 2 teaspoons of ground coriander
- 2 tablespoons of brown sugar
- 2 tablespoons of apple cider vinegar
- 1 tablespoon of mustard
- 1 tablespoon of canned tomato paste

Instructions:

- In a bowl, add the coriander, dry mustard, salt, black pepper, and garlic powder. Mix well.
- Rub and coat the spice mixture over the turkey thighs.
- Add the turkey thighs to your Instant Pot and add in the beer.
- Lock the lid and cook at high pressure for 45 minutes.
- When the cooking is done, quick release the pressure and remove the lid.
- Transfer the turkey thighs to a plate and shred using forks. Set aside.
- Press "Saute" function on your Instant Pot and allow the liquid to simmer until reduced to about half.
- Stir in the brown sugar, apple cider vinegar, mustard, and tomato paste until smooth. Cook for 1 minute, stirring occasionally.
- Return the turkey and give a good stir.

Nutrition information per serving:

- Calories: 406
- Fat: 20.1g
- Carbohydrates: 3g
- Dietary Fiber: 0g
- Protein: 44.7g

6. Extraordinary Honey Garlic Chicken

Time: 25 minutes

Servings: 4

Freestyle SmartPoints: 9

Ingredients:

- 4 to 6 bone-in, skinless chicken thighs
- 1/3 cup of honey
- 4 garlic cloves, minced
- ½ cup of low-sodium soy sauce
- ½ cup of sugar-free ketchup
- ½ teaspoon of dried oregano
- 2 tablespoons of parsley, chopped
- 1 tablespoon of sesame seed oil
- 1 teaspoon of salt
- 1 teaspoon of black pepper
- ½ tablespoon of toasted sesame seeds, for garnish

Instructions:

- In a bowl, add the honey, garlic, soy sauce, ketchup, oregano, and parsley Mix until well combined and set aside.
- Season the chicken thighs with salt and pepper.
- Press "Saute" function and add the sesame oil.
- Once the oil is hot, add the chicken thighs and cook for 3 minutes on both sides.
- Add the honey garlic sauce to your Instant Pot.
- Lock the lid and cook at high pressure for 20 minutes.
- When the cooking is done, naturally release the pressure for 5 minutes and quick release any remaining pressure.
- Transfer the chicken to serving plate and spoon the sauce over. Serve and enjoy!

Nutrition information per serving:

- Calories: 360
- Fat: 10g
- Carbohydrates: 35g
- Dietary Fiber: 6g
- Protein: 32g

7. **Refreshing Duck Confit**

Time: 2 hours

Servings: 4

Freestyle SmartPoints: 3

Ingredients:

- 4 duck legs
- 2 tablespoons of olive oil
- 1 tablespoon of salt
- 4 sprigs fresh thyme
- 4 garlic cloves, crushed
- 2 bay leaves, torn in half
- ¼ teaspoon of black peppercorns, crushed
- ¼ teaspoon of allspice berries, crushed

Instructions:

- Season the duck legs with salt, bay leaves, peppercorns, and allspice.
- Press "Saute" function on your Instant Pot and add the olive oil.
- Once the oil is hot, add the duck legs and cook until golden brown on both sides.
- Add the garlic and thyme on top of the duck.
- Lock the lid and cook at high pressure for 40 minutes. You don't need to add any additional liquid as the duck legs contain enough moisture to create steam.
- When the timer beeps, quick release the pressure and remove the lid. Flip the duck legs over.
- Lock the lid and cook at high pressure for 30 minutes.
- When the cooking is done, naturally release the pressure and remove the lid.
- Remove the duck legs and allow to cool.
- Serve and enjoy!

Nutrition information per serving:

- Calories: 194
- Fat: 11.5g
- Carbohydrates: 0g
- Dietary Fiber: 0g
- Protein: 21.8g

8. Exquisite Orange Duck and Gravy

Time: 1 hour and 30 minutes   Servings: 4   Freestyle SmartPoints: 5

Ingredients:

- 4 duck legs
- 2 tablespoons of avocado oil
- 1 yellow onion, chopped
- 1 celery rib, chopped
- 1 large carrot, chopped
- 8 garlic cloves, crushed
- 1 tablespoon of tomato paste
- ½ cup of chicken stock
- 1 teaspoon of orange zest
- ¼ cup of orange juice
- 2 tablespoons of Italian parsley, chopped
- 1 dried bay leaf
- 1 fresh thyme sprig
- ½ teaspoon of herbes de Provence
- 1 teaspoon of salt
- 1 teaspoon of black pepper

Instructions:

- In a small bowl, add the salt, black pepper, and herbes de Provence. Mix well.
- Sprinkle the seasonings over the duck legs.
- Press "Saute" function on your Instant Pot and add 1 tablespoon of avocado oil.
- Add the onions, celery, and carrots. Cook for 3 to 5 minutes or until the vegetables has softened, stirring occasionally.
- Add the garlic cloves and tomato paste. Cook for 30 seconds or until fragrant, stirring occasionally. Pour in the chicken stock to the pot.
- Stir in the orange juice, orange zest, parsley, bay leaf, and thyme. Turn off "Saute" function. Place the seasoned dug legs on top of the vegetables.
- Lock the lid and cook at high pressure for 45 minutes.
- When the cooking is done, naturally release the pressure for 20 minutes and remove the lid.
- Carefully remove the duck legs and discard the thyme sprig and bay leaf.
- Use an immersion blender to puree the contents of the Instant Pot until smooth and thick. Adjust the seasoning as needed.
- Heat a large cast-iron skillet over medium-high heat. Once the skillet is hot, add 1 tablespoon of avocado oil and duck legs. Cook for 2 to 3 minutes on both sides or until golden brown and crispy.
- Place the duck legs onto serving plates and spoon the gravy over. Serve!

Nutrition information per serving: Calories: 183, Fat: 5.6g, Carbohydrates: 9.5g, Dietary Fiber: 1.8g, Protein: 23.2g

Fish and Seafood Recipes

1. <u>Gorgeous Lemon-Shrimp Risotto with Vegetables and Parmesan</u>

Time: 25 minutes   Servings: 4   Freestyle SmartPoints: 4

Ingredients:

- 1 ½ cup of Arborio rice
- 1 pound of shrimp, peeled and deveined
- ½ cup of Parmigiano-Reggiano, shredded
- 2 teaspoons of olive oil
- 1 cup of fresh spinach
- 1 bunch of asparagus, sliced
- 3 ½ cup of chicken stock
- ½ cup of dry white wine
- 3 garlic cloves, minced
- ½ white onion, chopped
- 1 tablespoon of parsley, chopped
- ½ lemon, juiced
- 1 tablespoon of butter
- 1 teaspoon of salt
- 1 teaspoon of black pepper

Instructions:

- Press "Saute" function on your Instant Pot and add the olive oil.
- Once the oil is hot and ready, add the asparagus and cook for 3 minutes or until softened, stirring constantly. Once done, remove the asparagus.
- Add the onions and garlic and cook until fragrant, stirring occasionally.
- Add the butter and rice to your Instant Pot. Stir for 1 to 2 minutes or until the rice is coated in butter.
- Stir in the white wine, chicken stock, and cheese. Season with salt and black pepper. Lock the lid and cook at high pressure for 8 minutes.
- When the cooking is done, quick release the pressure and remove the lid.
- Press "Saute" function and add the shrimp, spinach, and asparagus.
- Cook for about 4 minutes or until the shrimp is pink and the spinach has wilted, stirring occasionally. Turn off "Saute" function. Drizzle with fresh lemon juice and sprinkle with parsley. Serve and enjoy!

Nutrition information per serving:

- Calories: 440
- Fat: 12g
- Carbohydrates: 48g
- Dietary Fiber: 4g
- Protein: 29g

2. Nourishing Garlic Butter Salmon and Asparagus

Time: 9 minutes

Servings: 3

Freestyle SmartPoints: 4

Ingredients:

- 1 pound of salmon fillets, cut into 3 equal pieces
- 1 pound of asparagus, cut into bite-sized pieces
- ¼ cup of lemon juice
- 3 tablespoons of butter
- 1 ½ tablespoon of garlic, minced
- 1 teaspoon of salt
- ¼ teaspoon of red pepper flakes
- 2 cups of water

Instructions:

- Lay 3 large pieces of foil on a flat surface.
- Place 1 salmon piece on each foil.
- Spread ½ tablespoon of garlic on each piece of salmon.
- Divide and place the asparagus equally between the three salmon pieces.
- Sprinkle salt and red pepper flakes on top of each salmon fillet.
- Add 1 tablespoon of butter on each salmon fillet.
- Tightly wrap the foil and make sure no steam can escape.
- Add 2 cups of water and a trivet to your Instant Pot.
- Place the foil packets on top of the trivet.
- Lock the lid and press "Steam" function and set for 4 minutes.
- When the cooking is done, quick release the pressure and remove the lid.
- Remove the foil packets and unopen. Transfer the contents to a plate.
- Serve and enjoy!

Nutrition information per serving:

- Calories: 343
- Fat: 21.2g
- Carbohydrates: 8.9g
- Dietary Fiber: 3.8g
- Protein: 33.2g

3. <u>Pleasant Fish and Potato Chowder</u>

Time: 30 minutes

Servings: 8

Freestyle SmartPoints: 4

Ingredients:

- 2 ½ cups of fish stock or water
- 1 ½ pounds of tilapia, cut into bite-sized pieces
- 1 pound of potatoes, chopped
- 1 cup of celery, chopped
- 1 cup of onions, chopped
- 6 bacon slices, chopped
- 1 ½ cup of unsweetened coconut cream
- 3 tablespoons of butter
- ½ teaspoon of garlic powder
- 1 teaspoon of salt
- 1 teaspoon of black pepper

Instructions:

- Press "Saute" function on your Instant Pot and add the bacon. Cook the bacon until brown and crispy.
- Remove the bacon and set aside.
- Add the butter, onions, and celery. Cook until the onions have softened, stirring frequently.
- Add the fish stock, tilapia pieces, salt, pepper, garlic powder, bacon and coconut cream to your Instant Pot. Give a good stir.
- Lock the lid and cook at high pressure for 10 minutes.
- When the cooking is done, naturally release the pressure and remove the lid.
- Use a potato masher to mash the potatoes until broken down. You can leave chunks if you prefer.
- Serve and enjoy!

Nutrition information per serving:

- Calories: 348
- Fat: 22.5g
- Carbohydrates: 13.3g
- Dietary Fiber: 2.9g
- Protein: 25g

4. <u>Soy-Free Asian Salmon</u>

Time: 7 minutes

Servings: 2

Freestyle SmartPoints: 3

Ingredients:

- 2 salmon fillets
- 1 tablespoon of coconut oil
- 1 tablespoon of brown sugar
- 3 tablespoons of coconut aminos
- 2 tablespoons of maple syrup
- 1 tablespoon of parsley, chopped
- 1 teaspoon of paprika
- ¼ teaspoon of ginger
- 1 teaspoon of sesame seeds
- 1 teaspoon of salt
- 1 teaspoon of black pepper

Instructions:

- Press "Saute" function on your Instant Pot and add the coconut oil.
- Once the oil is hot, add the brown sugar and stir until the sugar has dissolved.
- Stir in the paprika, ginger, coconut aminos, and maple syrup.
- Add the salmon fillets to your Instant Pot and season with salt and pepper.
- Lock the lid and cook at low pressure for 2 minutes.
- When the cooking is done, naturally release the pressure for 5 minutes and quick release any remaining pressure.
- Remove the lid and transfer the salmon fillets to a plate.
- Spoon and pour some of the broth over the salmon.
- Sprinkle the fillets with sesame seeds and garnish with parsley
- Serve and enjoy!

Nutrition information per serving:

- Calories: 378
- Fat: 17.8g
- Carbohydrates: 20.8g
- Dietary Fiber: 0g
- Protein: 34.5g

5. <u>**Traditional Lemon Garlic Salmon**</u>

Time: 10 minutes

Servings: 2

Freestyle SmartPoints: 2

Ingredients:

- 1 ½ pounds of frozen salmon fillets
- ¼ cup of lemon juice
- ¾ cup of fish stock or water
- 1 lemon, thinly sliced
- 1 tablespoon of coconut oil
- 2 tablespoons of mixed herbs
- 1 teaspoon of garlic powder
- 1 teaspoon of salt
- 1 teaspoon of black pepper

Instructions:

- Add the lemon juice, fish stock, and mixed herbs to your Instant Pot.
- Place a steamer rack in Instant Pot.
- Drizzle the salmon fillets with coconut oil and season with garlic powder, salt, and black pepper.
- Place the salmon on the steamer rack and place lemon slices on top.
- Lock the lid and cook at high pressure for 7 minutes.
- When the cooking is done, quick release the pressure and remove the lid.
- Serve and enjoy!

Nutrition information per serving:

- Calories: 539
- Fat: 28.8g
- Carbohydrates: 3.3g
- Dietary Fiber: 0.9g
- Protein: 58.5g

6. <u>Decorated Salmon, Broccoli, and Potatoes</u>

Time: 6 minutes

Servings: 2

Freestyle SmartPoints: 2

Ingredients:

- 2 (4-ounce) salmon fillet
- 1 medium head of broccoli, chopped into florets
- 1 potato, chopped into cubes
- 1 shallot, chopped
- 2 garlic cloves, minced

- 3 tablespoons of butter
- 1 tablespoon of coconut oil
- ½ cup of fish stock
- 1 tablespoon of parsley, chopped
- 1 teaspoon of salt
- 1 teaspoon of black pepper

Instructions:

- Drizzle the coconut oil over the salmon fillet and season with salt and pepper
- Press "Saute" function on your Instant Pot and add the butter.
- Once the butter has melted, add the shallot and cook until softened, stirring occasionally.
- Add the garlic and cook for 1 minute or until fragrant.
- Add the broccoli, potatoes, and parsley to your Instant Pot. Cook for 2 minutes, stirring occasionally.
- Add ½ cup of fish stock and a steaming rack to your Instant Pot.
- Place the salmon fillets on top of the rack.
- Lock the lid and cook at high pressure for 4 minutes.
- When the cooking is done, naturally release the pressure and remove the lid.
- Transfer the salmon fillet to a plate along with the broccoli and potato mixture.
- Serve and enjoy!

Nutrition information per serving:

- Calories: 467
- Fat: 31.8g
- Carbohydrates: 21.4g
- Dietary Fiber: 3.1g
- Protein: 27.1g

7. <u>Wonderful in Taste Fish Taco Bowls</u>

Time: 15 minutes

Servings: 4

Freestyle SmartPoints: 3

Fish Ingredients:

- 3 (6-ounce) cod fillets
- 1 tablespoon of olive oil
- ½ teaspoon of salt
- ½ teaspoon of black pepper
- 1 cup of water

Slaw Ingredients:

- ½ cup of green cabbage, grated
- 1 large carrot, peeled and grated
- 2 tablespoons of fresh orange juice
- 2 dashes of sriracha sauce
- ¼ cup of cilantro, freshly chopped
- ¼ cup of low-fat mayonnaise
- 1 medium avocado, peeled and diced
- 2 Roma tomatoes, chopped
- ½ large lime, juice
- 1 teaspoon of ground cumin
- 1 teaspoon of garlic salt

Instructions:

- In a large bowl, add all the slaw ingredients and stir until well combined.
- Add 1 cup of water and a trivet to your Instant Pot.
- Place a steamer basket on top of the trivet.
- Season the cod fillets with salt and pepper and drizzle olive oil.
- Place the cod fillets onto steamer basket.
- Lock the lid and cook at high pressure for 3 minutes.
- When the cooking is done, quick release the pressure and remove the lid.
- Distribute the slaw into serving bowls and add the cod fillet.
- Serve and enjoy!

Nutrition information per serving:

- Calories: 284
- Fat: 19.1g
- Carbohydrates: 13.4g
- Dietary Fiber: 4.8g
- Protein: 17g

8. __Wholesome Clam Chowder__

Time: 30 minutes

Servings: 6

Freestyle SmartPoints: 5

Ingredients:

- 3 (6.5-ounce) cans of chopped clams, juice reserved
- 4 slices of bacon, chopped
- 3 tablespoons of butter
- 1 onion, chopped
- 2 celery stalks, chopped
- 1 ½ pounds of potatoes, chopped
- 1 1/3 cup of heavy cream
- 1 tablespoon of cornstarch
- ¼ teaspoon of dried thyme
- 1 garlic clove, minced
- 1 ½ teaspoon of salt
- ¼ teaspoon of black pepper

Instructions:

- Press "Saute" function and add the chopped bacon to your Instant Pot. Cook the bacon until no more fat, but not crispy.
- Add the butter, onion, celery, and thyme. Cook for 4 minutes or until the onions are translucent, stirring occasionally.
- Add the garlic, salt, and black pepper. Cook for 1 minute or until fragrant, stirring frequently.
- Stir in the potatoes and clam juice.
- Lock the lid and cook at high pressure for 5 minutes.
- When the cooking is done, quick release the pressure and remove the lid.
- Use a potato masher and mash the potatoes.
- Press" Saute" function and stir in the clams and heavy cream.
- Add the cornstarch and cook until thickened. Adjust the seasoning as needed.
- Serve and enjoy!

Nutrition information per serving:

- Calories: 386
- Fat: 25.7g
- Carbohydrates: 32.7g
- Dietary Fiber: 4.9g
- Protein: 8.8g

Vegan and Vegetarian Recipes

1. Indian-Inspired Pickled Potatoes

Time: 15 minutes

Servings: 4

Freestyle SmartPoints: 3

Ingredients:

- 5 potatoes, boiled and cubed
- 4 tablespoons of olive oil
- 1 bay leaf
- 5 cloves
- 1 tablespoon of coriander seeds, pounded
- 1 tablespoon of cumin seeds
- 1 tablespoon of mango pickle
- 2 teaspoons of dried fenugreek leaves
- 1 teaspoon of dry pomegranate powder
- ½ teaspoon of turmeric powder
- ½ teaspoon of red chili powder
- 1 teaspoon of salt

Instructions:

- Press "Saute" function on your Instant Pot and add 2 tablespoons of olive oil.
- Once the oil is hot, add the cumin seeds, coriander seeds, cloves, and bay leaf. Allow simmering for a few seconds.
- Add the dry spices and mix them well.
- Add the remaining 2 tablespoons of olive oil and pickle. Stir the mixture well.
- Add the potatoes and coat them with the spice mixture.
- Lock the lid and cook at high pressure for 2 minutes.
- When the cooking is done, quick release the pressure and remove the lid.
- Serve and enjoy!

Nutrition information per serving:

- Calories: 304
- Fat: 14.3g
- Carbohydrates: 41.8g
- Dietary Fiber: 6.4g
- Protein: 4.5g

2. <u>Satisfying Vegan Quinoa Burrito Bowls</u>

Time: 25 minutes   Servings: 4   Freestyle SmartPoints: 3

Ingredients:

- 1 teaspoon of olive oil
- ½ red onion, chopped
- 1 sweet bell pepper, chopped
- 1 cup of quinoa, rinsed well
- 1 cup of salsa

- 1 cup of water
- 1 (15-ounce) can of black beans, drained and rinsed
- ½ teaspoon of salt
- 1 teaspoon of ground cumin

Topping ingredients (optional):

- Avocado slices
- Guacamole
- Fresh cilantro
- Green onions, chopped

- Salsa
- Lime wedges
- Lettuce, shredded

Instructions:

- Press "Saute" function on your Instant Pot and add the olive oil.
- Once the oil is hot, add the onions and pepper and cook for 5 minutes or until softened, stirring constantly.
- Add the cumin and salt and cook for an additional minute.
- Turn off "Saute" function on your Instant Pot.
- Add the quinoa, salsa, water, and black beans to your Instant Pot. Stir until well combined.
- Lock the lid and cook at low pressure for 12 minutes.
- When the cooking is done, naturally release the pressure and remove the lid.
- Fluff the quinoa with a fork and spoon into serving bowls.
- Top with your desired toppings.
- Serve and enjoy!

Nutrition information per serving:

- Calories: 562
- Fat: 5.5g
- Carbohydrates: 101.2g

- Dietary Fiber: 20.9g
- Protein: 30.4g

3. <u>Signature Curried Chickpea Stuffed Acorn Squash</u>

Time: 30 minutes   Servings: 2   Freestyle SmartPoints: 5

Ingredients:

- 2 cups of chickpeas, soaked in water for 30 minutes
- ¼ cup of brown rice washed and soaked in water for 30 minutes
- 2 cups of vegetable stock
- 1 small acorn squash, halved and deseeded
- 1 tablespoon of olive oil
- ½ teaspoon of cumin seeds
- ½ cup of red onions, chopped
- 4 garlic cloves, minced
- ½-inch ginger, minced
- 1 green chili, minced
- ¼ teaspoon of turmeric
- ½ teaspoon of garam masala
- ½ teaspoon of dry mango powder amchur
- 2 tomatoes, chopped
- ½ teaspoon of fresh lime juice
- 1 cup of rainbow chard or spinach, chopped
- ½ teaspoon of salt
- ¼ teaspoon of cayenne pepper

Instructions:

- Add the olive oil to your Instant Pot and press "Saute" setting.
- Add the cumin seeds and cook for 1 minute or until fragrant, stirring frequently.
- Add the onions, garlic, ginger, and chili. Cook for 5 minutes or until translucent, stirring frequently.
- Add the seasoning and stir for a couple of seconds.
- Add the tomatoes, lime juice, and rainbow chard or spinach. Cook for 5 minutes, stirring occasionally.
- Add the remaining ingredients except for the acorn squash to your Instant Pot and stir until well combined.
- Place a steamer basket or a trivet to your Instant Pot and place the acorn squash on top. Lock the lid and cook at high pressure for 17 minutes.
- When the cooking is done, naturally release the pressure and remove the lid.
- Carefully remove the steamer basket and stir the chickpea rice stew.
- Fill the squash with the chickpea rice mixture. Serve and enjoy!

Nutrition information per serving:

- Calories: 518
- Fat: 8g
- Carbohydrates: 97g
- Protein: 20g

4. <u>Terrific Vegan Sloppy Joes</u>

Time: 30 minutes

Servings: 8

Freestyle SmartPoints: 3

Ingredients:

- 1 cup of green/brown lentils
- 1 cup of red lentils
- 3 cups of water
- 1 large onion, chopped
- 1 red bell pepper, chopped
- 1 tablespoon of olive oil
- 2 tablespoons of apple cider vinegar
- 2 tablespoons of maple syrup
- 1 (28-ounce) can of crushed tomatoes
- 3 tablespoons of tomato paste
- 2 tablespoons of vegan Worcestershire sauce
- 1 teaspoon of salt
- 1 tablespoon of ground cumin
- 1 teaspoon of dried oregano

Instructions:

- Press "Saute" function on your Instant Pot and add the olive oil.
- Once the oil is hot, add the onion, bell pepper, and salt. Cook for 3 minutes or until softened, stirring frequently.
- Add the cumin and oregano and cook for 1 minute.
- Add the tomato paste and cook for 2 minutes, stirring to coat.
- Add the remaining ingredients and stir until well combined.
- Lock the lid and cook at high pressure for 13 minutes.
- When the cooking is done, allow for a natural release and remove the lid.
- Stir everything again and adjust the seasoning as needed.
- Serve over toasted hamburger buns.

Nutrition information per serving:

- Calories: 259
- Fat: 3.1g
- Carbohydrates: 47.3g
- Dietary Fiber: 5.4g
- Protein: 14.4g

5. <u>Mexican-Style Corn on the Cob with Hemp-Lime Sauce</u>

Time: 30 minutes

Servings: 4

Freestyle SmartPoints: 2

Ingredients:

- 4 ear corns, shucked and rinsed
- ½ cup of unsweetened coconut milk
- 2 tablespoons of hemp hearts
- 2 tablespoons of nutritional yeast
- 1 tablespoon of all-purpose flour
- 1 garlic clove, peeled
- ¼ teaspoon of cayenne pepper
- ¼ teaspoon of salt
- 1 tablespoon of fresh lime juice

Instructions:

- Place a trivet or a steaming basket inside your Instant Pot.
- Add 1 ½ cup of water and a trivet or steamer basket in your Instant Pot.
- Lock the lid and cook at high pressure for 4 minutes.
- When the cooking is done, quick release the pressure and remove the lid. Set the corn aside.
- In a blender, add the coconut milk, hemp hearts, nutritional yeast, flour, garlic, cayenne pepper, and salt. Blend until smooth.
- Pour into a saucepan and cook over medium-high heat, stirring constantly. Alternatively, you can add to your Instant Pot and cook at high pressure for 1 minute.
- Stir in the lime juice to the sauce.
- Drizzle the sauce over the corn.
- Serve and enjoy!

Nutrition information per serving:

- Calories: 190
- Fat: 4.6g
- Carbohydrates: 33.6g
- Dietary Fiber: 4.7g
- Protein: 9.3g

6. <u>Great Tasting Sweet Potatoes</u>

Time: 30 minutes

Servings: 4

Freestyle SmartPoints: 5

Ingredients:

- 4 raw sweet potatoes
- 2 cups of water

Instructions:

- Rinse and scrub the sweet potatoes
- Add 2 cups of water and a trivet to your Instant Pot.
- Place the potatoes on top of the trivet.
- Lock the lid and cook at high pressure for 18 minutes.
- When the cooking is done, naturally release the pressure.
- Carefully remove the lid and set the potatoes aside.
- Serve and enjoy!

Nutrition information per serving:

- Calories: 57
- Fat: 1g
- Carbohydrates: 15g
- Dietary Fiber: 2g
- Protein: 1g

7. To-Die-For Brussel Sprouts with Shallots

Time: 15 minutes

Servings: 8

Freestyle SmartPoints: 3

Ingredients:

- 2 pounds of Brussel sprouts, trimmed
- 1 or 2 shallots, finely chopped
- 1 tablespoon of olive oil
- ¼ cup of orange juice
- 2 tablespoons of maple syrup
- 1 teaspoon of salt
- 1 teaspoon of black pepper

Instructions:

- Press "Saute" function on your Instant Pot and add the olive oil.
- Once the oil is hot and ready, add the shallots and cook until brown and crispy, stirring occasionally.
- Turn off "Saute" function on your Instant Pot.
- Add the Brussel sprouts, orange juice, maple syrup, salt, and pepper in your Instant Pot.
- Lock the lid and cook at high pressure for 4 minutes.
- When the cooking is done, quick release the pressure and remove the lid.
- Stir until the Brussel sprouts are covered with the shallots and sauce.
- Serve and enjoy!

Nutrition information per serving:

- Calories: 65
- Fat: 2g
- Carbohydrates: 12g
- Dietary Fiber: 3g
- Protein: 3g

Rice and Grains Recipes

1. Lebanese Hashweh Ground Beef and Rice

Time: 30 minutes   Servings: 6   Freestyle SmartPoints: 5

Ingredients:

- 2 tablespoons of olive oil
- ¼ cup of pine nuts
- 1 cup of onions, sliced
- 1 tablespoon of garlic, minced
- 1 pound of ground beef
- ¼ teaspoon of ground cardamom
- 1 ½ teaspoon of ground allspice
- 1 teaspoon of ground cinnamon
- ¼ teaspoon of ground nutmeg
- 1 cup of basmati rice, rinsed and drained
- 1 teaspoon of salt
- 1 teaspoon of ground black pepper
- 1 cup of water
- ¼ cup of cilantro, chopped

Instructions:

- Press "Sauté" function on your Instant Pot and add the olive oil.
- Once the oil is hot and ready, add the pine nuts and cook for 1 to 2 minutes, stirring frequently.
- Add the minced garlic and onions. Stir well and cook until lightly browned.
- Add the ground beef and cook until brown, breaking up the ground beef with a wooden spoon.
- Add all the spices and stir well.
- Add the rice and 1 cups of water.
- Lock the lid and cook at high pressure for 4 minutes.
- When the cooking is done, naturally release the pressure for 10 minutes and quick release the remaining pressure.
- Fluff the rice with a fork and sprinkle with cilantro. Serve and enjoy!

Nutrition information per serving:

- Calories: 341
- Fat: 13.5g
- Carbohydrates: 27.7g
- Dietary Fiber: 1.1g
- Protein: 26.2g

2. <u>Tastiest Mexican Black Beans and Rice</u>

Time: 30 minutes

Servings: 4

Freestyle SmartPoints: 4

Ingredients:

- 1 (15-ounce) can of black beans, rinsed and drained
- 1 cup of brown rice
- 1 ½ cup of chicken broth
- ¾ cup of picante sauce

- 1 bay leaf
- 1 teaspoon of cumin
- 1 teaspoon of garlic salt
- 1 lime, juice

Toppings:

- Sour cream
- Tortilla chips

- Grated cheese
- Sliced avocados

Instructions:

- Add the black beans, brown rice, chicken broth, picante sauce, bay leaf, cumin, garlic salt, and lime juice to your Instant Pot.
- Lock the lid and cook at high pressure for 22 minutes.
- When the cooking is done, naturally release the pressure for 10 minutes and quick release the remaining pressure.
- Carefully remove the lid and discard the bay leaf.
- Stir the black beans and rice again and add more sauce as needed.
- Ladle into bowls and top with preferred toppings.
- Serve and enjoy!

Nutrition information per serving:

- Calories: 228
- Fat: 1.2g
- Carbohydrates: 44.4g
- Dietary Fiber: 8g
- Protein: 9.9g

3. <u>Kheema Pulao (Indian Meat and Rice)</u>

Time: 30 minutes   Servings: 6   Freestyle SmartPoints: 4

Pulao Ingredients:

- 2 teaspoons of ghee
- 1 red onion, thinly sliced
- 1 tablespoon of ginger, minced
- 1 tablespoon of garlic, minced
- 1 pound of lean ground beef

- 1 ½ teaspoon of salt
- 1 ½ cup of water
- 1 ½ cup of basmati rice
- 1 cup of frozen peas

Spices Ingredients:

- 1 teaspoon of cumin seeds
- 5 whole cloves
- 5 whole peppercorns

- 1 cinnamon stick, broken into pieces
- 3 teaspoons of garam masala

Instructions:

- Press "Saute" function on your Instant Pot and add the ghee.
- Once the ghee is hot, add the spices and cook for 30 seconds, stirring frequently.
- Add the garlic and ginger and cook for 30 seconds, stirring frequently.
- Add the ground beef and cook until lightly brown, stirring frequently and breaking up all the clumps.
- Add the onions, rice, salt, and water and stir until well combined.
- Lock the lid and cook at high pressure for 4 minutes.
- When the cooking is done, naturally release the pressure for 10 minutes and quick release the remaining pressure.
- Remove the lid and stir in the frozen peas.
- Serve and enjoy!

Nutrition information per serving:

- Calories: 354
- Fat: 6.6g
- Carbohydrates: 43.3g
- Dietary Fiber: 2.4g
- Protein: 27.9g

4. Sensational Chicken and Rice

Time: 25 minutes   Servings: 6   Freestyle SmartPoints: 3

Ingredients:

- 1 pound of boneless, skinless chicken thighs
- 1 tablespoon of avocado oil
- 3 small shallots, chopped
- 3 carrots, chopped
- 1 cup of mushrooms, sliced
- 2 garlic cloves, minced
- 1 ½ cup of white jasmine rice, rinsed and drained
- 1 ½ cup of chicken stock
- 2 tablespoons of fresh thyme leaves, chopped
- 1 teaspoon of salt
- 1 teaspoon of black pepper

Instructions:

- Press "Saute" function on your Instant Pot and add the avocado oil.
- Season the chicken thighs with salt and pepper.
- Once the oil is hot, add the chicken thighs and cook for 5 minutes per side.
- Remove the chicken and set aside.
- Add 1/3 cup of chicken stock to deglaze your Instant Pot. Scrape the bits with a wooden spoon.
- Add the shallots, mushroom, and carrots, and cook for 3 minutes, stirring frequently.
- Add the garlic and cook for 1 minute, stirring frequently.
- Add the chicken stock, rice, thyme and stir until well combined.
- Place the chicken thighs on top of the mixture.
- Lock the lid and cook at high pressure for 10 minutes.
- When the cooking is done, naturally release the pressure and remove the lid.
- Remove the chicken and shred using 2 forks.
- Return the chicken to your Instant Pot and stir.
- Serve and enjoy!

Nutrition information per serving:

- Calories: 347
- Fat: 6.5g
- Carbohydrates: 43.8g
- Dietary Fiber: 1.9g
- Protein: 26.5g

5. Scrumptious Mexican Rice

Time: 18 minutes

Servings: 12

Freestyle SmartPoints: 4

Ingredients:

- 2 tablespoons of avocado oil
- ¼ cup of onions, chopped
- 4 garlic cloves, minced
- 2 cusp of white rice
- 1 teaspoon of salt
- ¾ cups of crushed tomatoes
- 2 ½ cups of chicken stock
- ½ teaspoon of cumin
- ½ teaspoon of garlic powder
- ½ teaspoon of smoked paprika
- ¼ cup of cilantro, chopped

Instructions:

- Press "Saute" function on your Instant Pot and add the avocado oil.
- Once the oil is hot, add the onions and garlic. Cook for 3 minutes or until browned, stirring occasionally.
- Add the white rice and stir the rice until well coated with the oil, garlic, and onions.
- Add the chicken stock, crushed tomatoes, cilantro, cumin, smoked paprika, garlic powder, and salt.
- Lock the lid and cook at high pressure for 8 minutes.
- When the cooking is done, naturally release the pressure for5 minutes and quick release the remaining pressure.
- Remove the lid. Take a fork and lightly fluff the rice through.
- Serve and enjoy!

Nutrition information per serving:

- Calories: 510
- Fat: 14.2g
- Carbohydrates: 80.3g
- Dietary Fiber: 2.9g
- Protein: 13.6g

Soups, Stews, and Broths Recipes

1. Lovely Curry Cauliflower and Broccoli Soup

Time: 30 minutes   Servings: 8   Freestyle SmartPoints: 3

Ingredients:

- 1 large cauliflower head, chopped
- 1 large broccoli head, chopped
- 1 red bell pepper, chopped
- 1 green bell pepper, chopped
- 4 sweet potatoes, chopped
- 1 onion, finely chopped
- 2 garlic cloves, minced
- 2 cups of unsweetened coconut milk
- 2 cups of vegetable broth
- 1 tablespoon of coconut oil
- 2 tablespoons of yellow curry powder
- 1 teaspoon of cumin
- 1 teaspoon of dried thyme
- ½ teaspoon of cayenne pepper
- 1 teaspoon of salt
- 1 teaspoon of black pepper

Instructions:

- Press "saute" setting on your Instant Pot and add the coconut oil.
- Once the oil is hot and ready, add the onions and cook until translucent, stirring frequently.
- Add the garlic and cook for 1 minute or until fragrant.
- Add the cauliflower, broccoli, and red bell pepper. Cook for an additional minute, stirring occasionally.
- Add the remaining ingredients except for the coconut milk in your Instant Pot.
- Close the lid and cook at high pressure for 3 minutes.
- When the cooking is done, quick release the pressure and remove the lid.
- Stir in the coconut milk and adjust the seasoning as needed. Serve and enjoy!

Nutrition information per serving:

- Calories: 264
- Fat: 16.7g
- Carbohydrates: 26.4g
- Dietary Fiber: 7.2g
- Protein: 6.5g

2. Flavorful Chicken Tortilla-Less Soup

Time: 30 minutes

Servings: 8

Freestyle SmartPoints: 2

Ingredients:

- 1 ½ pounds of boneless, skinless chicken breasts
- 2 (10-ounce) cans of diced tomatoes and green chilies
- 1 (14.5-ounce) cans of chicken broth
- 2 zucchinis, chopped
- 1 ¾ cups of low-fat coconut cream
- 2 chipotle peppers in adobo sauce
- 2 teaspoons of adobo sauce
- 1 medium onion, chopped
- 2 teaspoons of garlic powder
- 1 teaspoon of onion powder
- 1 teaspoon of cumin
- 2 teaspoon of chili powder
- 1 teaspoon of dried oregano
- 1 teaspoon of smoked paprika
- 1 teaspoon of salt

Instructions:

- Add all the ingredients except for the coconut cream into your Instant Pot.
- Close and seal the lid.
- Cook at high pressure for 20 minutes.
- When the cooking is done, naturally release the pressure for 10 minutes and quick release any remaining pressure.
- Remove the chicken and chop into pieces.
- Return the cubed chicken to your Instant Pot and stir in the coconut cream.
- Serve and enjoy!

Nutrition information per serving:

- Calories: 169
- Fat: 3.1g
- Carbohydrates: 7.4g
- Dietary Fiber: 1.9g
- Protein: 27.3g

3. <u>Curried Carrot Red Lentil Soup</u>

Time: 35 minutes   Servings: 4   Freestyle SmartPoints: 3

Ingredients:

- 2 teaspoons of olive oil
- 1 cup of onions, chopped
- 1 tablespoon of ginger, grated
- 1 tablespoon of curry powder
- 2 cups of baby carrots, peeled and diced
- 4 cups of vegetable broth
- ¾ cups of dried red lentils rinsed well
- 1 teaspoons of salt
- ¼ teaspoon of ground black pepper

Instructions:

- Press "saute" function on your Instant Pot and add the olive oil.
- Once the oil is hot and ready, add the onions and cook until translucent, stirring frequently.
- Add the ginger and curry powder and cook for 30 seconds, stirring frequently.
- Add the carrots, vegetable broth, red lentils, salt, and black pepper. Stir until well combined.
- Lock the lid and cook at high pressure for 10 minutes.
- When the cooking is done, quick release the pressure and remove the lid.
- Use an immersion blender to puree the soup until smooth.
- Adjust the seasoning as needed.
- Serve and enjoy!

Nutrition information per serving:

- Calories: 209
- Fat: 4.4g
- Carbohydrates: 27.7g
- Dietary Fiber: 12.5g
- Protein: 14.8g

4. Scrumptious Sausage Italian Lentil and Barley Soup

Time: 25 minutes   Servings: 12   Freestyle SmartPoints: 2

Ingredients:

- 2 tablespoons of olive oil
- 1 pound of Italian sausage
- 1 ½ cup of dry lentils, rinsed
- 1 cup of kale, stemmed and finely chopped
- 1/3 cup of pearl barley
- 4 carrots, peeled and chopped
- 1 tablespoon of tomato paste
- 2 celery stalks, chopped
- 1 cup of onions, chopped

- 2 garlic cloves, minced
- 1 tablespoon of Italian seasoning
- ¼ teaspoon of red pepper flakes
- 1 teaspoon of salt
- 1 teaspoon of black pepper
- 5 cups of chicken stock
- 2 (15-ounce) can of crushed tomatoes
- ¼ cup of parsley, chopped
- 2 tablespoons of cider vinegar

Instructions:

- Press "saute" function on your Instant Pot and add the olive oil.
- Once the oil is hot and ready, add the Italian sausage and cook until no longer pink, breaking into smaller pieces with a spoon as you cook.
- Add the onions, celery, and carrots. Cook for 3 to 4 minutes or until the vegetables has softened.
- Stir in the garlic, tomato paste, Italian seasoning, parsley, red pepper flakes, and salt.
- Add the diced tomatoes, cider vinegar, pearl barley, beef stock, and lentils. Stir until well combined.
- Close the lid and cook at high pressure for 10 minutes.
- When the cooking is done, naturally release the pressure for 10 minutes and quick release any remaining pressure.
- Remove the lid and stir in the kale. Serve and enjoy!

Nutrition information per serving:

- Calories: 303
- Fat: 13.6g
- Carbohydrates: 28.8g

- Dietary Fiber: 11.4g
- Protein: 16.7g

5. Delectable Curry Pumpkin

Time: 20 minutes   Servings: 6   Freestyle SmartPoints: 4

Ingredients:

- 1 onion, chopped
- 2 teaspoons of olive oil
- 2 tablespoons of butter
- 3 tablespoons of all-purpose flour
- 2 tablespoons of curry powder
- 5 cups of vegetable broth
- 4 cups of pumpkin puree
- 1 ½ cups of low-fat coconut cream
- 2 tablespoons of soy sauce
- ½ tablespoon of brown sugar
- 1 teaspoon of lemon juice
- ½ teaspoon of lemon zest
- ¼ teaspoon of cayenne pepper
- ½ teaspoon of salt
- ½ teaspoon of black pepper

Instructions:

- Press "saute" function on your Instant Pot and add the olive oil.
- When the oil is hot and ready, add the onions and cook until softened.
- Remove and set aside.
- Melt the butter in your Instant Pot and stir in the flour and curry powder until smooth.
- Continue to stir until the mixture begins to bubble.
- Gradually stir in the vegetable broth.
- Add the pumpkin, onions, soy sauce, brown sugar, salt, and black pepper into your Instant Pot.
- Close the lid and cook at high pressure for 3 minutes.
- When the cooking is done, quick release the pressure and remove the lid.
- Stir in the coconut cream.
- Use an immersion blender and blend until smooth.
- Stir in the lemon juice and lemon zest. Serve and enjoy!

Nutrition information per serving:

- Calories: 307
- Fat: 21.7g
- Carbohydrates: 24.4g
- Dietary Fiber: 7.3g
- Protein: 8.5g

6. __Hearty Golden Lentil and Spinach Soup__

Time: 35 minutes

Servings: 4

Freestyle SmartPoints:

Ingredients:

- 2 teaspoons of olive oil
- 1 cup of onions, chopped
- 1 cup of carrots, chopped
- ½ cup of celery, chopped
- 4 garlic cloves, minced
- 2 teaspoons of ground cumin
- 1 teaspoon of ground turmeric
- 1 teaspoon of dried thyme
- 1 teaspoon of salt
- ¼ teaspoon of black pepper
- 1 cup of dry brown lentils, rinsed
- 4 cups of vegetable broth
- 6 cups of baby spinach

Instructions:

- Press "saute" function on your Instant Pot and add the olive oil.
- When the oil is hot and ready, add the onions, carrots, and celery. Cook until tender, stirring occasionally.
- Add the garlic, cumin, turmeric, thyme, salt, and black pepper. Cook for 1 minute, stirring constantly.
- Add the lentils and pour in the vegetable broth. Stir until well combined.
- Lock the lid on your Instant Pot and cook at high pressure for 12 minutes.
- When the cooking is done, quick release the pressure and remove the lid.
- Stir in the spinach until wilted.
- Serve and enjoy!

Nutrition information per serving:

- Calories: 98
- Fat: 4g
- Carbohydrates: 9.3g
- Dietary Fiber: 2.6g
- Protein: 7g

7. <u>**Delicious Italian Farmhouse Vegetable Soup**</u>

Time: 25 minutes

Servings: 4

Freestyle SmartPoints: 0

Ingredients:

- 1 tablespoon of olive oil
- 1 onion, chopped
- 2 celery sticks, sliced
- 2 carrots, peeled and sliced
- 6 mushrooms, sliced
- 4 porcini mushrooms, sliced
- 4 garlic cloves, minced
- ½ long red chili, sliced
- 2 cups of kale, stemmed and chopped
- 1 zucchini, chopped
- 1 cup of tomatoes, chopped
- 4 cups of vegetable stock
- 1 tablespoon of lemon juice
- 1 teaspoon of lemon zest
- 1 teaspoon of salt
- 1 teaspoon of black pepper

Instructions:

- Press "saute" function on your Instant Pot and add the olive oil.
- Once the oil is hot and ready, add the onion, salt, celery, and carrots. Cook for 2 minutes, stirring occasionally.
- Add the mushrooms, chili, and garlic. Cook for 1 minute, stirring occasionally.
- Add the remaining ingredients and stir until well combined.
- Lock the lid and cook at high pressure for 10 minutes.
- When the cooking is done, naturally release the pressure for 10 minutes and quick release any remaining pressure. Carefully remove the lid.
- Serve and enjoy!

Nutrition information per serving:

- Calories: 106
- Fat: 4.4g
- Carbohydrates: 15.1g
- Dietary Fiber: 3.3g
- Protein: 4.1g

8. <u>Creamy Cauliflower Soup</u>

Time: 30 minutes   Servings: 5   Freestyle SmartPoints: 2

Ingredients:

- 2 tablespoons of olive oil
- 1 onion, chopped
- 2 garlic cloves, minced
- 2 carrots, shredded
- 1 large head of cauliflower, chopped
- 1 cup of coconut cream
- 2/3 cup of mozzarella cheese, grated
- 1/3 cup of parmesan cheese, grated
- 2 cups of vegetable broth
- ¼ cup of butter
- ¼ cup of all-purpose flour
- 1 tablespoon of parsley
- 1 teaspoon of salt
- 1 teaspoon of black pepper

Instructions:

- Press "saute" setting on your Instant Pot and add the butter.
- Once the butter has melted, add the onions and cook until tender and golden.
- Add the garlic and cook for 1 minute.
- Add the carrots, cauliflower, vegetable broth, salt, and black pepper.
- Close the lid and cook at high pressure for 5 minutes.
- When the cooking is done, naturally release the pressure for 5 minutes and quick release any remaining pressure.
- Remove the lid from your Instant Pot.
- In a saucepan over medium-high heat, melt ¼ cup of butter.
- Stir in the ¼ cup of flour and stir until the mixture thickens and turns golden brown.
- Add the mozzarella cheese, parmesan cheese, and coconut cream in your Instant Pot and stir until melted.
- Add the flour mixture to the soup and stir until thickened.
- Garnish with parsley and adjust the seasoning as needed. Serve and enjoy!

Nutrition information per serving:

- Calories: 405
- Fat: 31.3g
- Carbohydrates: 22.3g
- Dietary Fiber: 6.6g
- Protein: 14.1g

9. **Supreme Taco Soup**

Time: 30 minutes   Servings: 10   Freestyle SmartPoints: 0

Ingredients:

- 1 ½ pound of ground turkey breast
- 1 large onion, chopped
- 1 tablespoon of olive oil
- 2 tablespoons of package Hidden Valley ranch dressing
- 2 tablespoons of taco seasoning mix
- 4 cups of chicken broth
- 1 (15-ounce) can of pinto beans
- 1 (15-ounce) can of hot chili beans
- 1 (15-ounce) can of whole kernel corns
- 1 (15-ounce) can of stewed tomatoes, Mexican flavor
- 1 (15-ounce) can of stewed tomatoes, any flavor
- 1 teaspoon of garlic powder
- 1 teaspoon of salt
- 1 teaspoon of black pepper

Instructions:

- Press "saute" function on your Instant Pot and add the ground turkey.
- Cook until the turkey is browned, stirring frequently.
- Add the olive oil and onions and cook for 5 minutes or until onions have softened.
- Add the remaining ingredients to your Instant Pot.
- Lock the lid and cook at high pressure for 15 minutes.
- When the cooking is done, quick release the pressure and remove the lid.
- Stir the soup again and adjust the seasoning as needed.
- Serve and enjoy!

Nutrition information per serving:

- Calories: 249
- Fat: 3g
- Carbohydrates: 39g
- Dietary Fiber: 8g
- Protein: 19g

10. Yummy Tomato Spinach Soup

Time: 20 minutes

Servings: 6

Freestyle SmartPoints: 1

Ingredients:

- 1 onion, chopped
- 2 garlic cloves, minced
- 2 carrots, grated
- 2 tablespoons of olive oil
- 1 pound of fresh spinach
- 1 (28-ounce) can of crushed tomatoes
- 1 ½ cups of chicken broth
- 2 teaspoons of dried basil
- 1 teaspoon of salt
- 1 teaspoon of black pepper
- 1 (5-ounce) can of evaporated milk

Instructions:

- Press "saute" setting on your Instant Pot and add the olive oil.
- Once the oil is hot, add the onions and carrots and cook until softened, stirring occasionally.
- Add the garlic and cook for 1 minute or until fragrant.
- Add the remaining ingredients except for the spinach and evaporated milk.
- Lock the lid and cook at high pressure for 15 minutes.
- When the cooking is done, naturally release the pressure for 10 minutes and quick release any remaining pressure.
- Remove the lid and carefully stir in the evaporated milk and spinach.
- Serve and enjoy!

Nutrition information per serving:

- Calories: 169
- Fat: 7.1g
- Carbohydrates: 20g
- Dietary Fiber: 6.8g
- Protein: 8.6g

11. **Flavorsome Chunky Beef, Cabbage, and Tomato Soup**

Time: 30 minutes   Servings: 7   Freestyle SmartPoints: 3

Ingredients:

- 1 pound of ground beef
- 1 onion, chopped
- 2 celery stalks, chopped
- 2 carrots, chopped
- 1 (28-ounce) can of diced tomatoes
- 5 cups of green cabbage, chopped
- 4 cups of beef stock
- 2 bay leaves
- 1 teaspoon of garlic powder
- 1 teaspoon of salt
- 1 teaspoon of black pepper

Instructions:

- Press "saute" function on your Instant Pot and add the olive oil.
- When the oil is hot, add the ground beef and cook until brown.
- When the ground beef has browned, add the onions, celery, and carrots and cook for 4 minutes or until softened.
- Add the tomatoes, cabbage, beef stock, and bay leaves.
- Lock the lid and cook at high pressure for 20 minutes.
- When the cooking is done, naturally release the pressure and remove the lid.
- Remove the bay leaves.
- Serve and enjoy!

Nutrition information per serving:

- Calories: 181
- Fat: 6g
- Carbohydrates: 14g
- Dietary Fiber: 2g
- Protein: 15.5g

12. Unique Loaded Baked Potato Soup

Time: 25 minutes

Servings: 6

Freestyle SmartPoints: 7

Ingredients:

- 2 pounds of potatoes
- 5 bacon slices, chopped
- ¼ cup of butter
- ¼ cup of flour
- 4 cups of milk
- ½ cup of sour cream
- ½ cup of cheddar cheese, grated
- 3 green onions, diced
- 1 teaspoon of bouillon chicken base
- 1 teaspoon of salt
- ½ teaspoon of black pepper

Instructions:

- Press "saute" function on your Instant Pot and add the bacon bits.
- Cook the bacon until brown and crispy. Once done, remove the bacon and set aside. Turn off "saute" function.
- Add 1 cup of water and a trivet inside your Instant Pot.
- Place the potatoes on top of the trivet.
- Lock the lid and cook at high pressure for 10 minutes.
- When the cooking is done, quick release the pressure and remove the lid.
- Remove the potatoes and set aside.
- Remove the water and discard the trivet.
- Press "saute" setting on your Instant Pot and add the butter.
- Once the butter has melted, add 1 tablespoon of flour and stir until begins to bubble. Add the milk and bouillon and start to whisk.
- Stir in the sour cream, cheddar cheese, diced onions, and bacon.
- Smash the potatoes with a potato masher and stir the potatoes into the soup.
- Add salt and black pepper to the soup. Serve and enjoy!

Nutrition information per serving:

- Calories: 439
- Fat: 25g
- Carbohydrates: 37.5g
- Dietary Fiber: 4g
- Protein: 17.5g

13. Exquisite Broccoli Cheese Soup

Time: 15 minutes   Servings: 6   Freestyle SmartPoints: 2

Ingredients:

- ¼ cup of butter
- 1 onion, finely chopped
- 2 cups of carrots, chopped
- 2 garlic cloves, minced
- ¼ cup of flour
- 3 cups of vegetable stock
- 6 cups of broccoli florets
- 1 teaspoon of paprika
- 1 teaspoon of Dijon mustard
- 1 ½ cups of Monterey jack cheese, shredded
- 1 ½ cups of sharp cheddar cheese, shredded
- ½ cup of milk
- ½ cup of coconut cream
- 1 teaspoon of salt
- 1 teaspoon of black pepper

Instructions:

- Press "saute" setting on your Instant Pot and add the butter.
- When the butter is melted, add the onions and carrots and cook for 3 minutes or until onions are translucent.
- Stir in the garlic and flour and cook for 1 minute.
- Stir in the broth and continue to stir until flour lumps are gone.
- Add the broccoli and vegetable stock to your Instant Pot.
- Lock the lid and cook at high pressure for 8 minutes.
- When the cooking is done, quick release the pressure and remove the lid.
- Stir in the paprika, Dijon mustard, salt, and black pepper until well incorporated.
- Stir in the cheeses until fully melted.
- Once the cheese has melted, add the milk and coconut cream.
- If you prefer, use an immersion blender to blend the soup until reached your desired consistency. Serve and enjoy!

Nutrition information per serving:

- Calories: 228
- Fat: 14.6g
- Carbohydrates: 18.5g
- Dietary Fiber: 5.1g
- Protein: 7.2g

Appetizers and Side Dishes Recipes

1. <u>Cheesy Rotel Queso Dip</u>

Time: 20 minutes   Servings: 11   Freestyle SmartPoints: 2

Ingredients:

- 2 cups of ground Italian sausage
- 1 (10-ounce) can of Rotel tomatoes with chiles, diced and drained
- 2 jalapenos, seeded and diced
- 1 poblano pepper, diced
- 1 cup of onions, minced
- 3 garlic cloves, minced
- 2 teaspoons of canola oil
- ¼ cup of cilantro, chopped

- 2 cups of shredded reduced-fat sharp Cheddar, Sargento
- ½ cup of low sodium chicken broth
- 1 cup of skim milk
- 3 tablespoons of cornstarch
- 1 lime, juice and zest
- ½ teaspoon of ground cumin
- 1 teaspoon of ancho chili powder

Instructions:

- In a small bowl, mix ¼ cup of skim milk with 3 tablespoons of cornstarch. Set aside. Press "saute" function on your Instant Pot and add the canola oil.
- Once the oil is hot and ready, add the onions, garlic, poblano, and jalapeno. Cook until softened, about 5 to 7 minutes, stirring frequently.
- Turn off "saute" function on your Instant Pot.
- Add the chicken broth, sausage, tomatoes, and 1 cup of cheese to your Instant Pot. Lock the lid and cook at high pressure for 5 minutes.
- When the cooking is done, naturally release the pressure for 5 minutes and quick release the remaining pressure.
- Press "saute" function on your Instant Pot and stir in the remaining ingredients.
- Cook and stir until the cheese has completely melted. Serve and enjoy!

Nutrition information per serving:

- Calories: 92.5
- Fat: 4.6g
- Carbohydrates: 7g

- Dietary Fiber: 1g
- Protein: 6.5g

2. <u>Cabbage with Turkey Sausage</u>

Time: 10 minutes

Servings: 8

Freestyle SmartPoints: 2

Ingredients:

- 1 pound of Turkey sausage, sliced
- 1 large cabbage head, chopped
- 1 onion, chopped
- 3 garlic cloves, minced
- 2 teaspoons of sugar
- 2 teaspoons of balsamic vinegar
- 2 teaspoons of Dijon mustard
- 1 tablespoon of olive oil
- 1 teaspoon of salt
- 1 teaspoon of black pepper

Instructions:

- Press "Saute" function on your Instant Pot and add the olive oil.
- Once the oil is hot and ready, add the Turkey sausage and onions. Cook until slightly browned.
- Add the cabbage and remaining ingredients to your Instant Pot. Cook until the cabbage cooks down, stirring frequently.
- Turn off "Saute" function on your Instant Pot. Adjust the seasoning as needed.
- Serve and enjoy!

Nutrition information per serving:

- Calories: 220
- Fat: 17.9g
- Carbohydrates: 3g
- Dietary Fiber: 0.5g
- Protein: 11.3g

3. **Fit for a King Spinach Artichoke Macaroni and Cheese**

Time: 25 minutes   Servings: 6   Freestyle SmartPoints: 6

Ingredients:

- 2 tablespoons of olive oil
- 1 large onion, finely chopped
- 10 garlic cloves, minced
- 1 can of artichoke hearts, drained and roughly chopped
- 1 pound of pasta
- 12-ounces of baby spinach
- 6 cups of vegetable broth
- 1 teaspoon of red pepper flakes

- 1 teaspoon of salt
- 1 teaspoon of black pepper
- 4-ounces of cream cheese softened
- ¼ cup of parmesan cheese, grated
- 1 cup of shredded low-fat mozzarella

Instructions:

- Press "saute" function on your Instant Pot and add the olive oil.
- Once the oil is hot and ready, add the onions and cook for 2 minutes or until translucent.
- Add the garlic and cook for 1 minute or until fragrant, stirring frequently.
- Add the artichoke hearts and cook for another minute.
- Add the pasta and 5 cups of vegetable broth.
- Lock the lid and cook at high pressure for 4 minutes.
- When the cooking is done, quick release the pressure and remove the lid.
- Stir in the remaining vegetable broth. If the pasta looks watery, don't add.
- Press "saute" function on your Instant Pot and fold in the baby spinach. Cook until the spinach wilts.
- Stir in the cream cheese, mozzarella, and parmesan.
- Season with red pepper flakes, salt, and black pepper. Stir everything until everything is well combined and the cheese has melted. Serve and enjoy!

Nutrition information per serving:

- Calories: 509
- Fat: 18g
- Carbohydrates: 65g

- Dietary Fiber: 4g
- Protein: 22g

4. <u>Smoky Baked Beans</u>

Time: 45 minutes

Servings: 12

Freestyle SmartPoints: 2

Ingredients:

- 1 pound of dried navy beans, soaked overnight and rinsed
- 1 tablespoon of salt
- 8 slices of bacon, cut into ½-inch pieces
- 1 large onion, chopped
- 2 ½ cups of chicken stock
- ½ cup of molasses
- ½ cup of ketchup
- ¼ cup of packed brown sugar
- 1 teaspoon of dry mustard
- ½ teaspoon of black pepper

Instructions:

- Press "saute" function on your Instant Pot and add the bacon bits. Cook until brown and crispy, stirring occasionally.
- Remove the bacon bits and place on paper towels.
- Add the onions to the bacon grease and cook until tender, about 3 minutes.
- Add the chicken stock, molasses, ketchup, brown sugar, dry mustard, salt, and black pepper to your Instant Pot. Stir until well combined.
- Stir in the soaked navy beans.
- Lock the lid and cook at high pressure for 35 minutes.
- When the cooking is done, naturally release the pressure for 10 minutes and quick release any remaining pressure. Remove the lid.
- Stir in the cooked bacon and press "saute" function. Simmer the beans, stirring occasionally, until the sauce reaches your desired consistency.
- Serve and enjoy!

Nutrition information per serving:

- Calories: 264
- Fat: 6.1g
- Carbohydrates: 40g
- Dietary Fiber: 9.5g
- Protein: 13.6g

5. <u>Classic Potato Salad</u>

Time: 10 minutes + 1 hour of refrigerating time

Servings: 8

Freestyle SmartPoints: 3

Ingredients:

- 6 medium russet potatoes, peeled and cubed
- 1 ½ cup of water
- 4 large eggs
- ¼ cup of onions, finely chopped
- 1 cup of fat-free mayonnaise
- 2 tablespoons of parsley
- 1 tablespoon of pickle juice
- 1 tablespoon of mustard
- ½ teaspoon of salt
- ½ teaspoon of black pepper

Instructions:

- Place a steamer basket inside your Instant Pot.
- Add the water, potatoes, and eggs.
- Lock the lid and cook at high pressure for 4 minutes.
- When the cooking is done, quick release the pressure and remove the lid.
- Remove the steamer basket from your Instant Pot and place the eggs in an ice bath.
- Allow the potatoes to cool. Peel and dice the cooled eggs.
- In a large bowl, combine the onions, mayonnaise, pickle juice, and mustard.
- Stir in the potatoes and eggs into the potato salad.
- Season with salt and black pepper. Refrigerate for 1 hour before serving.

Nutrition information per serving:

- Calories: 258
- Fat: 12.2g
- Carbohydrates: 32.7g
- Dietary Fiber: 3.9g
- Protein: 5.8g

6. <u>Contest-Winning Chili Con Carne</u>

Time: 20 minutes   Servings: 8   Freestyle SmartPoints: 8

Ingredients:

- 1 pound of ground beef
- 1 (28-ounce) can of whole peeled tomatoes, undrained
- 1 (14-ounce) can of black beans, rinsed and drained
- 1 (14-ounce) can of kidney beans, rinsed and drained
- 3 tablespoons of olive oil
- 1 large onion, finely chopped
- 1 red bell pepper, chopped
- 2 medium jalapenos, chopped
- 2 garlic cloves, minced
- 1 teaspoon of ground cumin
- 1 tablespoon of chili powder
- 1 teaspoon of dried oregano
- 1 ½ teaspoon of salt
- ½ teaspoon of black pepper

Instructions:

- Press "saute" function on your Instant Pot and add the olive oil.
- Once the oil is hot and ready, add the ground beef and cook until brown, breaking it into smaller pieces with a spoon.
- Add the onions, bell pepper, and jalapenos into your Instant Pot and cook for 3 minutes.
- Add the garlic, cumin, chili powder, oregano, salt, and black pepper. Cook for 1 minute, stirring occasionally.
- Add the Worcestershire sauce, tomatoes, water, and beans. Stir until well combined.
- Lock the lid on your Instant Pot and cook at high pressure for 10 minutes.
- When the cooking is done, naturally release the pressure for 10 minutes and quick release any remaining pressure.
- Press "saute" function and cook until the chili has thickened or reached your desired consistency. Serve and enjoy!

Nutrition information per serving:

- Calories: 519
- Fat: 10.3g
- Carbohydrates: 68.6g
- Dietary Fiber: 17g
- Protein: 40.4g

7. **Drive-Thru Tacos**

Time: 20 minutes   Servings: 4   Freestyle SmartPoints: 6

Ingredients:

- 1 pound of ground beef
- 1 tablespoon of Worcestershire sauce
- 1 tablespoon of olive oil
- 1 cup of beef broth
- 2 teaspoons of all-purpose flour
- 1 tablespoon of chili powder
- ¼ teaspoon of garlic powder
- ¼ teaspoon of onion powder
- ¼ teaspoon of dried minced onions
- 1 ½ teaspoon of ground cumin
- ¼ teaspoon of dried oregano
- ½ teaspoon of paprika
- 1 teaspoon of salt
- ½ teaspoon of black pepper
- A pinch of cayenne pepper
- Taco shells (for serving)

Instructions:

- Press "saute" function on your Instant Pot and add the olive oil.
- Once hot and ready, add the ground beef and cook until brown, stirring occasionally.
- Turn off "saute" function.
- Add the remaining ingredients in your Instant Pot. Stir until well combined.
- Lock the lid and cook at high pressure for 3 minutes.
- When the cooking is done, naturally release the pressure for 10 minutes and quick release any remaining pressure.
- Remove the lid and press "saute" function. Mix and allow to simmer until most of the liquid has reduced.
- Spoon the taco meat onto taco shells.
- Serve and enjoy!

Nutrition information per serving:

- Calories: 259
- Fat: 10.9g
- Carbohydrates: 2g
- Dietary Fiber: 0g
- Protein: 35.7g

8. <u>Fun to Eat Monkey Bread</u>

Time: 25 minutes   Servings: 8   Freestyle SmartPoints: 5

Ingredients:

- 3 ½ cups of all-purpose flour
- ¾ cups of sugar
- ¼-ounces of active dry variety yeast
- 1 teaspoon of salt
- 1 cup of low-fat milk
- ½ cup of unsalted butter softened
- 1 large egg, beaten
- 1 teaspoon of ground cinnamon
- ¼ teaspoon of ground nutmeg
- 1/8 teaspoon of cloves

Instructions:

- In a large bowl, add 1 ½ cup of all-purpose flour, ¼ cup of sugar, yeast, and salt. Mix well.
- Use an electric mixer and gradually beat in the milk and ¼ cup of butter.
- Add the egg and remaining flour and beat for 2 minutes.
- Turn the dough onto a floured counter and knead until smooth and elastic.
- Cover the dough with plastic wrap and allow to rest for 10 minutes.
- In a small bowl, add ¼ cup of melted butter.
- In a second bowl, add ½ cup of sugar, cinnamon, nutmeg, and cloves.
- Divide the dough into 4 quarters.
- Dip each dough quarter into the butter mixture and coat well with the sugar mixture.
- Place the biscuit pieces into a greased mini loaf pan.
- Add 1 cup of water and a trivet to your Instant Pot.
- Place the loaf pan on top of the trivet. Cover with a piece of aluminum foil.
- Lock the lid and cook at high pressure for 21 minutes.
- When the cooking is done, naturally release the pressure for 5 minutes and quick release any remaining pressure.
- Remove the lid and allow the bread to cool Serve and enjoy!

Nutrition information per serving:

- Calories: 398
- Fat: 13.3g
- Carbohydrates: 62.4g
- Dietary Fiber: 1.7g
- Protein: 7.9g

9. Perfect Little Smokies

Time: 10 minutes

Servings: 8

Freestyle SmartPoints: 2

Ingredients:

- 2 (12-ounce) packages of Cocktail Sausages
- 8-ounces of barbecue sauce
- ¼ cup of light brown sugar
- 1 tablespoon of white vinegar
- 1 tablespoon of honey
- 4-ounces of beer

Instructions:

- Add the sausages to your Instant Pot.
- Add the barbecue sauce, brown sugar, white vinegar, honey, and beer to the sausages. Stir until well combined.
- Lock the lid and cook at high pressure for 1minute.
- When the cooking is done, naturally release the pressure for 1 minute and quick release the remaining pressure.
- Press "Saute" in your Instant Pot. Cook and stir for 5 minutes to thicken the sauce.
- Serve and enjoy!

Nutrition information per serving:

- Calories: 363
- Fat: 24.2g
- Carbohydrates: 17.4g
- Dietary Fiber: 0.2g
- Protein: 16.6g

Desserts Recipes

1. <u>Secret Chocolate Cupcakes</u>

Time: 40 minutes   Servings: 8   Freestyle SmartPoints: 4

Cupcake Ingredients:

- 1 box of chocolate cake mix
- 1 (15-ounce) can of pumpkin
- ¼ cup of water

Frosting ingredients:

- ¼ cup of peanut butter
- 1 teaspoons of cocoa powder
- 2 tablespoons of maple syrup

Instructions:

- In a large bowl, add and mix all the cupcake ingredients.
- Fill silicone cupcake liners ¾ full. If you don't have silicone cupcake liners, you can use ramekins or heat-safe glass jars. Cover with aluminum foil.
- Add 1 ½ cups of water and a trivet inside your Instant Pot.
- Place the cupcakes on the trivet.
- Close the lid and cook at high pressure for 25 minutes.
- When the cooking is done, naturally release the pressure and remove the lid.
- Carefully remove the cupcakes and allow to cool.
- In a bowl, add and mix all the frosting ingredients until well combined.
- Spoon the frosting on top of the cupcakes.
- Serve and enjoy

Nutrition information per serving:

- Calories: 359
- Fat: 14.5g
- Carbohydrates: 57.2g
- Dietary Fiber: 3.7g
- Protein: 6.5g

2. Satisfying Blueberry Compote

Time: 20 minutes

Servings: 2

Freestyle SmartPoints: 4

Ingredients:

- 3 cups of frozen blueberries
- ¾ cups of sugar
- 2 tablespoons of lemon juice
- 2 tablespoons of cornstarch
- 2 tablespoons of water

Instructions:

- Add the blueberries, sugar, and lemon juice inside your Instant Pot. Stir until well combined.
- Lock the lid and cook at high pressure for 3 minutes.
- When the cooking is done, naturally release the pressure for 10 minutes and quick release any remaining pressure.
- In a small bowl, mix the cornstarch with the water.
- Press saute on your Instant Pot and stir in the cornstarch mixture until thickened.
- Place in a storage container and refrigerate for at least 3 hours.
- Serve and enjoy!

Nutrition information per serving:

- Calories: 440
- Fat: 0.9g
- Carbohydrates: 114.1g
- Dietary Fiber: 5.4g
- Protein: 1.9g

3. <u>**Elegant Blackberry Cobbler**</u>

Time: 20 minutes

Servings: 6

Freestyle SmartPoints: 6

Ingredients:

- 1 (12-ounce) package of fresh blackberries, washed and dry
- 8-ounces of white cake mix
- ¼ cup of butter
- 1 cup of water

Instructions:

- Grease an oven safe dish that will fit in your Instant Pot with nonstick cooking spray.
- Add the blackberries to the dish.
- In a bowl, using a pastry blender cut the butter into the cake mix until resembles crumbly texture.
- Spread the cake mixture over the blackberries.
- Tightly cover with aluminum foil.
- Add 1 cup of water and a trivet inside your Instant Pot.
- Place the oven safe dish on top.
- Lock the lid of your Instant Pot and cook at high pressure for 10 minutes.
- When the cooking is done, naturally release the pressure for 10 minutes and quick release any remaining pressure.
- Remove the lid and carefully remove the dish from your Instant Pot.
- Allow cooling for 10 minutes.
- Serve and enjoy!

Nutrition information per serving:

- Calories: 253
- Fat: 12.1g
- Carbohydrates: 34.9g
- Dietary Fiber: 3.4g
- Protein: 2.6g

4. Glorious Chocolate Chip Bundt Cake

Time: 40 minutes   Servings: 12   Freestyle SmartPoints: 6

Ingredients:

- 1 (16.5-ounces) of chocolate fudge cake mix
- 2 tablespoons of all-purpose flour
- 1 (3-ounce) package of chocolate dry pudding mix
- 1 cup of buttermilk
- ½ cup of warm water
- ¼ cup of unsweetened applesauce
- 2 tablespoons of coconut oil
- 1 teaspoon of vanilla extract
- 2 large eggs, beaten
- 1 cup of chocolate chips

Topping ingredients:

- 2 tablespoons of powdered sugar

Instructions:

- In a large bowl, add all the cake ingredients except for the chocolate chips and mix until well combined.
- Fold in the chocolate chips.
- Grease a bundt pan with nonstick cooking spray.
- Pour the cake batter into the greased bundt pan.
- Tightly cover the bundt pan with aluminum foil.
- Add 1 ½ cups of water and a trivet inside your Instant Pot.
- Place the bundt pan on top of the trivet and close the lid.
- Cook at high pressure for 25 minutes.
- When the cooking is done, quick release the pressure and remove the lid.
- Carefully remove the cake from your Instant Pot and allow to cool for 10 minutes. Sprinkle powdered sugar over the cake. Serve and enjoy!

Nutrition information per serving:

- Calories: 291
- Fat: 11.6g
- Carbohydrates: 42g
- Dietary Fiber: 1g
- Protein: 4.7g

5. Enticing Pumpkin Chocolate Chip Bundt Cake

Time: 35 minutes   Servings: 8   Freestyle SmartPoints: 8

Ingredients:

- 1 ½ cups of all-purpose flour
- 1 teaspoon of pumpkin pie spice
- 1 teaspoon of ground cinnamon
- 1/4 teaspoon of salt
- ½ teaspoon of baking soda
- ½ teaspoon of baking powder
- ½ cup of butter softened
- 1 cup of sugar
- 2 large eggs, beaten
- 1 cup of pumpkin puree
- ¾ cups of mini-chocolate chips

Instructions:

- In a bowl, add the flour, pumpkin pie spice, cinnamon, salt, baking soda, and baking powder. Mix well.
- In another bowl, beat the butter and sugar until fluffy.
- Mix in the eggs one at a time.
- Add the pumpkin and mix until well combined.
- Add the flour mixture and mix until well combined.
- Fold in the chocolate chips.
- Grease a 6-cup bundt pan with nonstick cooking spray.
- Spoon the batter into the bundt pan. Tightly cover with aluminum foil.
- Add 1 ½ cup of water and a trivet inside your Instant Pot.
- Put the bundt pan on the trivet.
- Close and lock the lid. Cook at high pressure for 25 minutes.
- When the cooking is done, naturally release the pressure for 10 minutes and quick release any remaining pressure.
- Carefully remove the lid and carefully remove the bundt pan.
- Allow cooling for 10 minutes. Serve and enjoy!

Nutrition information per serving:

- Calories: 395
- Fat: 17.8g
- Carbohydrates: 55.4g
- Dietary Fiber: 2.3g
- Protein: 5.7g

6. Delightful Banana Chocolate-Chip Mini Muffins

Time: 10 minutes   Servings: 16   Freestyle SmartPoints: 4

Ingredients:

- 1 cup of vanilla yogurt
- ½ cup of fat-free skim milk
- 1/2 cup of quick oats
- ½ teaspoon of vanilla extract
- 1 large egg, beaten
- 1 large bananas, mashed
- 1 ¼ cup of all-purpose flour
- ¼ cup of brown sugar
- 2 teaspoons of baking powder
- ½ teaspoon of salt
- ½ teaspoon of baking soda
- ½ cup of mini-chocolate chips, divided

Instructions:

- In a bowl, add the milk, vanilla yogurt, vanilla extract, and eggs. Mix until well combined.
- Add the quick oats, bananas, flour, brown sugar, baking powder, salt, and baking soda. Stir until well combined.
- Fold in the chocolate chips.
- Add 1 cup of water and a trivet inside your Instant Pot.
- Using a cookie scoop, fill silicone muffins with the batter.
- Layer the muffin cups inside your Instant Pot. (Note: You may need to cook the muffins in batches if any leftover batter.)
- Cover the muffin cups with aluminum foil to prevent water from resting on top.
- Close and seal your Instant Pot.
- Cook at high pressure for 8 minutes.
- When the cooking is done, naturally release the pressure and remove the lid.
- Check if the muffins are done using a toothpick.
- Remove the muffins and allow to cool. Serve and enjoy!

Nutrition information per serving:

- Calories: 107
- Fat: 2.5g
- Carbohydrates: 17.7g
- Dietary Fiber: 0.9g
- Protein: 3.3g

The Final Words

Thank you very much for downloading and reading this book about the Weight Watchers Program!

After reading this book, you got to know what the Weight Watchers program is, how to get started, how to stick with it, and 120 Weight Watchers Freestyle SmartPoints recipes using your Instant Pot! You also have a 2-week sample meal plan and tips for succeeding in this program. With all that, I am certain you will see positive results following this program.

Lastly, if you enjoyed this book, please take the time to review it on Amazon. Your honest feedback would be greatly appreciated.

Thank you, and the best of blessings on your weight loss journey!

CPSIA information can be obtained
at www.ICGtesting.com
Printed in the USA
BVHW051925250221
601128BV00008B/747